My Friends Walk Barefoot

Jim Humphreys, DVM

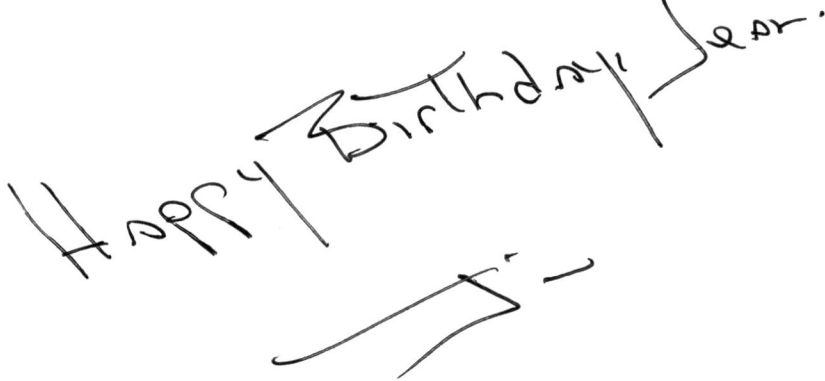

MY FRIENDS WALK BAREFOOT

My Friends Walk Barefoot
Copyright © 2022 by Jim Humphreys. All rights reserved.
ISBN: 978-1-387-81924-9

No part of this publication may be reproduced, stored by a retrieval system, or transmitted in any way by any means, electronic, mechanical, photocopy, recording, or otherwise without the prior permission of the author except as provided by USA copyright law.

All stories are based on true events.
A few names of characters have been changed.
This book was published in the United States of America.

Edited by Efrem Carrasco
Cover Design by Anna Hileman

Ladera Press
6 Cuates Canyon
Las Cruces, NM 88011
eldocjim@gmail.com

To Kay,

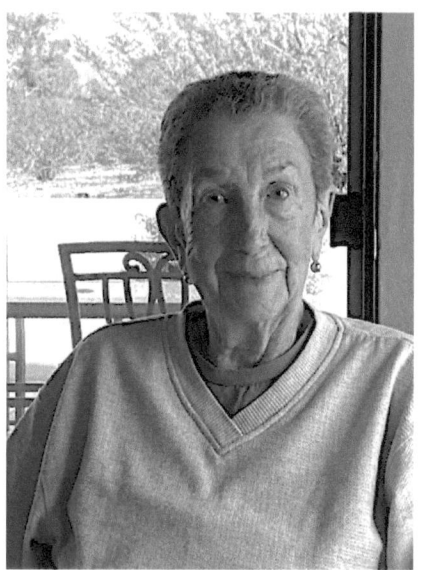

My mother-in-law, my writing teacher,
my inspiration, and my greatest fan.

MY FRIENDS WALK BAREFOOT

This is for Katy, JT, and Rob, whose enduring love and support is a continuous reminder of what a lucky man I am.

My love to Mike, my staff, to Jay, and to my clients and friends who provided the memories.

Thanks to my friends at the Desert Writers and our mentors: Ann, Paula, Leora, and Susan for their tough, critical evaluation of my writing.

Finally, my heartfelt thanks to Efrem Carrasco, my editor and my friend who reminded me on a weekly basis that, "This is quite a book, Jim."

Table of Contents

Preface..iv

Prologue...v

1. Jay and Flossy..1
2. Hearts..15
3. Tale of Two Dummies..27
4. A Lesson from Scrutch..45
5. Buttons..55
6. Yellow Magic...67
7. Lucky???...81
8. Banjo..95
9. Time for a Baby?..107
10. The Devil in the Sale Barn......................................120
11. Jay Meets Carrie..135
12. Hershey...147
13. Cowboy Jack...161
14. Funny How Things Turn Out.......................................173
15. Dancer..187
16. Ostrich Heaven..199
17. Brenda's Song...213
18. Rani..223
19. Rani Part II..237
20. Time to Say Goodbye...247

Epilogue...259

PREFACE

My Friends Walk Barefoot is an accumulation of stories based on actual events. In my forty years of practicing veterinary medicine, I experienced a multitude of adventures—some dangerous, others comical, and all of them memorable.

Although some of the names have been changed, the characters in this book are real, as are the laughs and tears we shared. Over the years, I have told my stories to family and friends at the supper table and other get-togethers. The response I have received has always been the same—"You need to write a book, Jim."

And so, here it is. I believe some of these stories will make you laugh, while others will make you cry. I hope you enjoy them.

Jim

PROLOGUE

He was loading something into a shiny white shell that covered the entire bed of his pickup when I drove into the parking lot of the animal clinic. He was tall and thin, with short hair and blue eyes.

"Excuse me, sir," I said as I approached him and extended my hand. "I'm Jim Humphreys." He looked at me with a wide smile and shook my hand.

"I'm Mark Cox. What can I do for you."

"Well, uh . . . I'm a third-year college student in a bit of a crisis," I said, in a voice that did little to disguise my embarrassment. He looked puzzled.

"You wanna tell me about it?" he asked. I couldn't believe he hadn't told me to get lost and walked away, but he stood there and waited for my answer.

"Well, you see," I continued, "I feel like I should have some idea by now as to what I want to do after I graduate." I sighed. "I don't . . . have any idea, that is. My sister's father-in-law is a veterinarian. She suggested I consider looking into veterinary medicine as a profession. I don't suppose, just maybe, you might need some help? Would you consider, maybe . . . letting me tag along with you for a while?"

Again, he smiled. It was a warm, confident, and compassionate smile that became a constant presence in our relationship. He opened the door to his pickup.

"We have a horse to go look at. Hop in."

He was my mentor. He was present at my wedding and my graduation from veterinary school. He led me down the path that would define a forty-year career. He is my dear friend.

Chapter 1

JAY AND FLOSSY

Jay dressed in a sleeveless tie-dye shirt, Bermuda shorts, and sandals. I wore a shirt, coveralls, and boots. We stepped into the pickup and drove off.

"So, where are we going?" Jay asked.

"We're going to see Flossy, Jane Washburn's spoiled little . . ."

"Did you say Floozy?"

"Flossy, Jay. Flossy," I repeated. "By the way, she has a bad habit of kicking and biting. Aren't you glad you decided to come along?" I asked with a devilish grin.

Over the years, I had a number of patients whose less than cooperative attitudes made treating them a challenge. Miss Flossy was at the top of that list.

I've also had the good fortune of having many good friends, and a few great ones. Jay remains at the top of the few.

Following graduation, I arrived in Roswell, a town of 45,000, at the foot of the mountains in southeastern New Mexico. My wife, Katy, had moved a few months ahead of me. Our one-bedroom rented house was cozy and attractive except for the old military-green linoleum that covered the floors throughout the house.

We decided it was time to look for a carpet. Our living room was top priority. A Sunday newspaper ad caught my eye.

15 by 15-foot, low pile carpet and pad.
Good condition. Fifty dollars. Call Jay.

I called the number listed. "Hi. Is this Jay? I'm calling about the ad in the paper. Do you still have that carpet?"

"Yes, this is Jay and yes, I still have the carpet." His voice was that of a man who was mellow . . . relaxed.

"Can you tell me what color it is?" I asked.

"Well, let me see." There was a long pause and then, "I guess I'd call it kinda . . . baby-shit yellow. You know what I mean?"

I was familiar with that hue, but had never heard it described in those terms. Katy and I didn't have any children, but I had nephews and had changed a few diapers.

"Yeah, I think so. When can I see it?" I asked.

"How about now?"

"Sounds great. I just moved here, Jay. Don't know the area. Where do I go?"

His directions were detailed and perfect. Jay waited to greet us. He was six feet tall, thin, and well-muscled. He wore blue jeans, a "Grateful Dead" t-shirt, and sandals. His blonde hair fell to his shoulders and his mustache, thick, but well-trimmed, extended down both cheeks to his chin. We stepped out of the car.

"Jay, I'm Jim Humphreys. This is my wife, Katy."

"Glad to meet you guys." He shook hands with both of us. "Come on in. My girlfriend and I just moved here from Dallas. She hates this carpet, so out it goes. I gotta admit it's not the prettiest color I've ever seen, but I think the price is right."

We walked into the living room. Katy and I looked at the carpet and then at each other. It was definitely…baby-shit yellow. "Do you have kids?" I asked.

"Who, me? Not that I know of. Why?"

"Oh, just asking." I turned to Katy. "What do you think, sweetie?"

After a few seconds passed, "Uh, sure. Looks great," she said.

"Well, okay. Sounds like we've got a deal," Jay said, excited to be rid of it.

I wrote a check for fifty dollars. Jay rolled up the carpet.

"What brought you guys to New Mexico?" he asked.

"Jim just graduated from veterinary school. He has a job with a local group," Katy said. "I'm an engineer. I work for U.S.D.A. What about you, Jay? What brought you here from the big city?"

"I've been asking myself that very question for a while now." He grinned. "You see, my grandfather and his brother founded a ranch on the west side of town back in the early 1900s. My grandfather died a few months ago and his brother is having a hard time handling the place on his own. It's a big ranch. He asked for my help. I was a teen in California during the sixties. You know, peace, love, drugs, and rock and roll. Closest I ever got to ranching was a worm farm I had in the back of my VW van. That was, until I smoked a little weed and fell asleep on the beach in Santa Monica one day. When I woke up, I was burned to a crisp. So were my worms."

Who would make that up, I thought. I really liked this guy.

"What did you do in Dallas, Jay?" I asked.

"I was a master welder working on a high-rise. I was making good money, too. Dallas is a bit crazy, but it sure beats the hell out of this place. By the way, how are you going to get this thing home?"

"Uh, I hadn't thought about that." I was embarrassed. Katy and I had driven to pick up this carpet in a Toyota Corolla.

"Aw, don't worry about it," Jay chuckled. "We can load it in my pickup and I'll follow you home."

I wasn't sure what to say. "Really? Uh, okay." We loaded the carpet and were on our way.

Jay and I laid the pad and the carpet in our living room. It fit almost perfectly. I searched for something other than a simple thank you. As usual, Katy came to the rescue. "How about joining us for lunch, Jay."

"Yeah. I'd like that. I'm kinda on my own this weekend. My girlfriend is back in Dallas packing the last of our things. She's not in a big hurry to move here. She's an interior decorator. Real artsy. Big city type. Don't think she's terribly excited about this ranching gig."

We sat around the card table that passed for a kitchen table, ate a plate of nachos, and drank the last few beers I had in the refrigerator. Katy and I enjoyed the company of our new friend.

1 – Jay and Flossy

When he got up to leave, he said, "I really want you guys to meet my girlfriend."

"We'd love to, Jay," Katy said. "What's her name?"

Dana was tall and thin with straight blonde hair that reached halfway down her back. Despite a few philosophical differences, she and Katy became great friends. Over the next year, we spent a lot of time together camping, dinners out, rafting down the creek that traversed the ranch, or just enjoying a Saturday afternoon sitting under the trees, sipping margaritas and grilling a rack of ribs.

It was Saturday evening. Jay and Dana arrived at six o'clock. Katy poured margaritas for herself and Dana as I passed Jay a beer and lit the grill. I prepared the steaks and then my pager rang. I had forgotten I was on call.

The message read, *Please call Mrs. Washburn. Flossy in trouble.* I reached for the phone.

"Dr. Humphreys," the trembling voice said. "Thank God you're on call. Flossy is really sick. I think she may have the colic."

"I'll be there in twenty minutes," I replied. "Keep her walking until I get there. Don't let her get down and roll, understand?" I hung up, looked at our guests, and shook my head. "Sorry, guys. I gotta go."

"What's up?" Jay asked, now on his second beer.

"Got an emergency, Jay. Wish I could put it off for a while, but I don't think this one can wait."

"I'll go with you," he said without hesitation.

"No, you don't want to do that. You stay here and cook the steaks. I should be back in an hour or so."

"The steaks can wait, right, girls?" Katy and Dana both held up their margaritas, smiled, and nodded.

"There you go," Jay said. "The sooner we take care of this minor inconvenience, the sooner we get back."

"If you insist. Let's go," I said.

Jane Washburn was in her mid-fifties, divorced, with no children. Her family consisted of Flossy, two dogs, a cat, three goats, and a few chickens. They all lived happily on a small farm on the outskirts of town at the end of a rocky road. Behind a modest little rock house was a two-acre field, completely fenced, with one gate wide enough for vehicle entrance.

We drove through the gate into Flossy's playground. Jane was walking Flossy just as I had instructed. She wore a bright pink robe with matching slippers and hair curlers. For the first time, Jay set eyes on Flossy, an average-sized donkey—600 pounds, four feet tall at the withers, that is, the top of her shoulders, with light grey hair and brown eyes. The halter and long lead rope that Jane led her by were a perfect match—also bright pink.

"You suppose she picked up the whole pink package at a garage sale?" Jay asked.

"Hi, Ms. Washburn," I said.

"Thank God you're here, Dr. Humphreys," she said. "I'm so worried about her. She's been kicking at her sides and trying to lie down."

"Well, let's have a look. I brought some help, ma'am. This is my friend, Jay." Jay smiled and nodded. She stared at my hippie friend, his

1 – *Jay and Flossy*

long hair, his shirt, his sandals, as if to say, why on earth would you bring him?

We approached Flossy. Normally erect, her ears lay back, flat against her head. Her nostrils flared and she began a series of rhythmic, emphatic snorts—she was not happy to see us.

I hesitated for a moment. Jay stood behind me. "Tell you what, Ms. Washburn," I said. "Why don't you let Jay hang onto her while I examine her a bit closer, okay?"

I looked over my shoulder at Jay. "You're kidding, right," he said with a disbelieving look on his face.

"I don't know, Dr Humphreys," Jane said. "You know she's pretty particular about people. She loves you, but I don't know about him," she said as she pointed a trembling forefinger at Jay. "You love Dr. Humphreys, don't you, Flossy?"

The truth was that Flossy didn't love anybody, even Jane, who would never admit that this sweet-looking little donkey was in fact, a real bitch.

"She'll be alright, Ms. Washburn," I said with a smile. After considerable thought, she reluctantly gave up the bright pink lead rope.

Jane looked directly into the donkey's eyes. "You be good, Flossy. You know Dr. Humphreys is a good man. He and his . . . friend are going to make you feel better, okay?"

I took the lead rope from Jane who discreetly stepped away as though distancing herself from a ticking time bomb.

"Watch her . . . closely," I whispered as I passed the rope to Jay who now seemed less enthusiastic.

"Don't worry, I will," he replied through clenched teeth.

We approached Flossy's left side. Jay's right hand took a firm hold of the lead rope, inches off her chin. Slowly, he laid his left hand across the top of her nose. He extended his thumb as though threatening to poke her in the eye should she give him cause.

The object of my exam was to listen for motility in Flossy's intestines, measure her heart rate, and evaluate the color of her gums—three critical physiological parameters that indicate whether a colic case is relatively minor or serious. An elevated heart rate accompanied by a lack of gut sounds and a bluish or a muddy color to the gums is a sure sign that a horse or donkey is in big trouble.

I ran my left hand slowly down Flossy's back. A general rule of horsemanship is to stay close to the shoulder and use a touch of the hand to let the animal know where you are—it decreases the chances of being kicked. With my right hand, I placed my stethoscope on the donkey's abdomen and as expected, she shot her back foot straight forward, narrowly missing a direct hit to my groin.

"You okay?" Jay asked.

"That was close," I said. "You might have had to finish this on your own. Hang on." Again, I placed the stethoscope on Flossy's belly. This time she allowed it. It was hard to hear anything over the pounding of my own heart, but the distinct gurgling sound of gas passing through her intestines was a good sign. I knew that her dissatisfaction could easily have raised her heart rate to well above normal and that any attempt to measure it might prove futile. I backed away.

1 – Jay and Flossy

Flossy looked at me and lifted her upper lip, exposing her front teeth, a gesture of total defiance. Unknowingly, she gave me the opportunity to evaluate the color of her gums. Like her halter and lead rope, they were a healthy bright pink.

"I think she's okay, Ms. Washburn. Her vital signs are good," I said. "A gallon of mineral oil in her belly and some pain killer should put her back on track."

"Whatever you say, Dr. Humphreys. You know Flossy and I trust you." She wiped her tears.

"A gallon of mineral oil in her belly? Just how do you intend to do that?" Jay whispered. There was growing concern in his voice.

"I have to pass a stomach tube through her nose and down her esophagus. Then we can pump the oil into her stomach."

"What! Are you nuts?" he exclaimed.

"Well, let's give it a shot. What's the worst that can happen," I said. "Have you got her?"

"Hell no, I don't got her. She's got me!" Jay was no longer whispering.

"Just don't make any sudden moves," I said. I walked to my truck and opened my mobile pharmacy, a fiberglass box which fit snuggly in the bed. I drew up ten milliliters of Banamine with a needle and syringe, my best option for alleviating the pain of colic. I emptied a gallon jug of mineral oil into a stainless-steel bucket, grabbed a ten-foot stomach tube, a stomach pump, and headed back.

Jay and Flossy both stood motionless. I set the bucket and pump down, laid the tube across the back of my neck and over my shoulders.

"Jay, I need you to move back toward her shoulder . . . very slowly," I said.

Without saying a word, he obeyed. I stepped up to Flossy and carefully extended my right hand out across the top of her nose. My left hand held the tip of the tube. I spoke in my softest voice. "Okay, girl, if you'll just be real still, I'm going to slip this tiny little tube up your nose and then . . . "

Without warning, Flossy leapt forward, jerking the lead rope from Jay's hand, knocking over the bucket, and spilling the oil. Jay wrapped both arms around the donkey's neck and held on tightly.

The fenced two acres were littered with mesquite bushes, prickly pear, and barrel cactus. They were particularly thick along the edge of the fence. Like the start of the Kentucky Derby, they were off, Flossy at full speed with Jay draped across her shoulders, his legs dragging on the ground. He tried unsuccessfully to skip over the cactus. I was in hot pursuit, following a trail of dust. Explicit obscenities poured from Jay's mouth, drowned out only by Jane's screams, "DON'T YOU HURT HER!"

Had Jay failed to close the gate, I might never have seen either of them again. As it was, the fenced field limited her path. She did, however, run the entire fence perimeter. She dragged Jay through the tallest mesquite bushes and thickest cactus she could find. His unprotected legs and feet were no match for New Mexico's finest thorny flora.

I continued the chase. Finally, Flossy's stylish pink lead rope wrapped itself around her front legs. It slowed her down just enough for Jay to get his feet on the ground and keep a firm hold of the rope. Flossy passed the only tree in the entire field. Jay dove for the base of the tree, threw the rope around the trunk, and held tight.

Flossy reached the end of her rope and frustrated by her loss of control of the situation, she bucked and kicked violently. Each time the donkey's feet became airborne, Jay frantically pulled on the rope. He drew her closer and closer until her nose and the trunk of the tree were one.

Jane's screams filled the air. "BE GOOD, FLOSSY!"

It took me a while, but I finally arrived at the base of the tree, huffing and puffing.

"Where the hell have you been!" Jay barked.

"Sorry, man," I squeezed out between breaths. "Don't let her go."

"I have no intention of letting her go!"

I lifted the syringe from my breast pocket. I squeezed the barrel of the syringe in the palm of my hand like a knife, removed the cover from the needle, and positioned my thumb firmly on the plunger. I stabbed the bucking beast in the side of her neck and delivered the full dose of Banamine deep into her muscle.

"Turn her loose," I yelled.

"What?" Jay looked stunned.

"I said, turn her loose!"

Reluctantly, Jay let go of the rope. The demonic donkey brayed and jerked on the rope until it finally came loose. She ran, bucking and kicking across the open field.

Jay stood and watched her go. The setting sun cast a crimson hue behind his silhouette. Dust and debris in the air added to the creepiness of his lacerated, bloody body. His hair was dusty and tangled. His arms, legs, t-shirt, and shorts were covered in blood. One sandal was partially torn from his foot. The other was missing.

"You just had to say something about putting that tube up her nose, didn't you," Jay said with disgust. "Why didn't you just shut up and do it!" He shook his head. "Can we go home now?"

I hadn't been able to finish my treatment plan. The mineral oil was an added precaution, but Flossy's intestinal motility was normal. I knew the Banamine would quickly control her pain. I considered our options and decided that another attempt at pumping mineral oil into her stomach was not likely to be successful, likely to get Jay and me killed, and unnecessary. I gathered the empty bucket, stomach tube, and pump.

"We've done what we can, Ms. Washburn. We're going home. Sorry I couldn't get her halter off," I said regretfully.

"Is she going to be okay, Dr. Humphreys?" Jane asked. Strangely, she was calm.

"She's gonna be just fine, Ms. Washburn. That painkiller I gave her should kick in pretty soon. Besides, she's too ornery to die."

She smiled, stepped forward, stood on her tiptoes, and placed a gentle kiss on my cheek. "I can always count on you, Dr. Humphreys. Thank you so much for taking care of my Flossy."

I helped Jay back to the pickup, dumped him in, and we drove away.

1 – Jay and Flossy

Back at the house, I washed up. "Jay, I'll get you some clean clothes," I yelled. "Leave the bloody ones outside the shower door. I'll throw them in the washer." I stepped onto the porch and lit the grill as he stepped into the shower.

I poured the wine. Jay took two ibuprofens followed by a sip of wine, raised his glass, and toasted, "Here's to Flossy. May she jump that fence and never come home."

Sunday morning, after a cup of coffee, I decided to call and check on my friend. "Dana? It's Jim. How's Jay?"

"Oh, he's okay, Jim. He's on the couch licking his wounds."

"Is he mad at me?"

"What?" she chuckled.

"I really wanna know. Is he mad at me?"

She talked away from the phone. "Hey, Jay! Jim wants to know if you're mad at him."

In the distance, I heard him say, "What?"

"Jim wants to know if you're mad at him," she repeated. After a long pause, he said something, soft, muffled, and difficult to understand.

"Jim? Jay said to tell you he doesn't get mad . . . He gets even."

IN THE BEGINNING.............

Chapter 2

HEARTS

Katy was not one to beat around the bush. We had only been married for a year, but having been high school sweethearts, she knew me very well.

"What's the matter?"

"Oh, it's nothing," I replied.

The truth was, she knew me better than I knew myself. "Don't give me that. What's up?"

I sighed. "I don't know. I'm getting spooked, I guess."

"About what?"

"About keeping up with the rest of my class. I got used to being the guy who set the curve back at UTEP (University of Texas El Paso). Now I'm surrounded by brainiacs. I feel like a sardine swimming in a pool of sharks. These are smart people, sweetie. I mean really smart."

"So are you," she said. "You wouldn't be in this pool if you weren't. You'd still be in that fishbowl back in El Paso wondering what to do with your biology degree. Don't worry about everybody else. Grow some teeth. Make some friends." She reached across the breakfast table, kissed me on the cheek, and smiled. "You're going to be just fine."

I finished my last piece of toast and followed it with a swallow of milk. "I better get dressed," I said as I pushed away from the table.

It was the '70s, a time of blue jeans and t-shirts, but the dress code at the College of Veterinary Medicine at Texas A&M University was strict. Women were required to wear a skirt or slacks and a blouse. We men wore dark shoes, white cotton slacks, a collared shirt, and tie. No scrubs allowed. We all wore a white zip-up smock with our name tag above the breast pocket.

I stood before the mirror tying my tie. Katy walked behind me and put her arms around my waist. "Why don't you join that study group? Gina says it's really helped Dan."

"I don't know Dan that well."

"Well, you should. He's your classmate and our neighbor, for Pete's sake." She shook her head. "I know you're no social butterfly, but maybe you need to work at it a bit."

Of course, she was right. I had been a veterinary student for over six months. I was a member of an elite group of young men and women who had worked hard to get where we were. Some of my classmates were starting a career they had dreamed of since they were old enough to talk. School counselors had reinforced how heavy the stress would be and how important it was for us to work as a team and support each other. "You all need to be friends. Good friends," they had said.

I put on my smock and brushed the lint off my shoulders. "How do I look?"

Katy handed me my backpack, straightened my tie, and kissed me. "You look great. I packed your lunch and put it in the zipper pocket behind your books." She helped me sling the backpack over my shoulders and patted me on the back. "I may be late getting home this afternoon. We're surveying today. You know what that means."

Katy was a graduate student in engineering. College Station, Texas was hot and humid, at times unbearable for humans, but a haven for crawling, squirming, and flying bugs . . . and ticks. A day in the field surveying meant I would be picking the ticks off her body when she got home.

"Promise me you'll make a friend today," Katy said with a smile.

"Yes ma'am," I said as I walked out the door.

Our first Monday morning class was Physiology. 125 students gathered in a large auditorium. Lab classes were in the afternoon. At that time, we were split into four groups assigned to separate smaller rooms.

Dr. Don Clark was our professor. A true genius, Dr. Clark completed his residency and board certification in cardiology at Baylor University Medical School in Houston. He was tall and thin, spoke softly, and wore a bowtie. He had a great sense of humor, but was demanding of us.

"Good morning, Ladies and Gents. Today, we're getting acquainted with electrocardiography. You know, that beeping squiggly line that races across a screen telling the ER doc that his patient is still alive." He smiled. "That simple little blip on the screen holds a world of secrets about what's happening microscopically in that amazing little muscle that pounds away, sixty times a minute, day and night, keeping us among the living. Let's get started."

He picked up the yardstick that he used for a pointer, turned on the slide projector, and directed our attention to the first slide, a picture of a normal E.C.G.

"Every beat of a living heart is governed by nerve impulses that can be recorded by a beautiful machine we call the electrocardiograph. What we see on the monitor attached to this fabulous recorder is a tight grouping of three waves that correspond to a single heartbeat. We call them the P-wave, the QRS-wave, and the T-wave." He pointed to the slide on the screen. "This is what we expect from a normal heart."

He went on to describe normal rhythm vs. arrhythmia. Missing P-waves, an enlarged or inverted T-wave, or a prolonged Q to T interval were all critical hints that what you heard with your stethoscope may not be a healthy heart after all. Over the next hour, he detailed the effects of oxygen deprivation, disease, drugs, and changes in electrolyte levels on "P, QRS and T."

"I realize we've just covered a lot of material," Dr. Clark said. "This afternoon's lab will help to tie it all up in a little bow. We'll all meet upstairs in the small theater . . . room 205. Be prepared to answer questions."

We filed out into the hallway. Most of my classmates were shaking their heads. I thanked God I wasn't the only one feeling overwhelmed.

After lunch, I hurried to room 205. I wanted to get there before anyone else arrived. If I could get a seat in the back row, maybe I would be better protected from the bombardment of Dr. Clark's questions.

I peeked through the door and saw a friendly face. Ronny Hooker had the same idea I did and was sitting in the back row. The room was a typical small theater with a capacity of 200. There were ten rows of seats, each row one step higher than the row before it. A single aisle of stairs in the center of the room climbed to the back row which was backed by a wall. The seats were wooden and uncomfortable.

At the front of the room were two stainless steel surgery tables. Each table held a dog laid flat on his back. Both had been anesthetized. A trained technician sat next to each table and monitored vital signs of the respective patient. The dogs were hooked up to an electrocardiograph and covered by a surgical drape with only the chest exposed. Their sternums had been split lengthwise and large steel retractors pulled apart the ribs, exposing their beating hearts. Cameras hung directly over the open chest cavities, the images shown on a large screen.

The practice of using live dogs for teaching purposes was accepted in the day. Most of the dogs acquired by the school were greyhounds that had been retired from the racetrack and were scheduled for immediate euthanasia. At the veterinary school, the dogs were well fed, well exercised with love and care. When their day to participate in the teaching process arrived, they were anesthetized by a trained technician, never to wake up after the procedure. Years passed and with the advent of pre-recorded video and canine rescue organizations, that practice was deemed inhumane and unnecessary and was abandoned. My class had the privilege of learning firsthand, what future generations of veterinary students would learn only from film and a textbook.

I climbed the steps of the center aisle to the back row and pointed to the seat next to Ronny. "Okay if I sit here, Ronny?"

"You bet, Jim. Gotta warn ya, though. It's hot up here. I don't think the air conditioner is working."

Ronny was about six feet tall, 180 pounds of solid muscle, a football star in high school. He had been offered several full-ride scholarships from division-one colleges. Pursuing a dream of being a veterinarian, he decided to forego football, get good grades, and try for veterinary school. He was one of only three students in our class who was accepted after two years of college instead of four, or more. Although I didn't know him well, Ronny struck me as a kind, unpretentious guy. He was soft spoken and always smiled. Over the following years, we became great friends.

I sat down and waited as the rest of the class began to file in. There were two screens on the wall behind the dogs. The top two thirds of each screen was the live video of an open chest and a beating heart. The bottom third showed the continuous corresponding E.C.G.

The room was full when Dr. Clark walked through the door. "Good afternoon, Ladies and Gents. We have a lot to cover, so let's get started." He pointed to one of the dogs. "This fine gentleman is Wile E. Coyote. He's a four-year old Greyhound with an athletic heart which you see here on the left screen. Next to him is Bear, a thirteen-year-old Labrador with a badly diseased heart." He pointed to the screen on the right. "Bear's owner has been treating his congestive heart failure for some time. He's been losing ground." He sighed and with genuine sadness in his voice, he said, "Mrs. Johnson brought him in this morning to be euthanized and graciously consented to give us some time with him prior to his demise. She did so hoping that what you learn here today will enable all of you, sometime in the future, to help other dogs who suffer with the same condition that Bear suffered." The room was silent. Dr. Clark continued, "Let us all give a genuine effort for the next hour as a way of paying our respect and giving our appreciation to these two guys who are giving us their all. Are we ready?"

He picked up his yardstick and turned toward the screens. "On our left, we see Sir Wile E.'s heart, a beautiful pear-shape, rich, healthy color, and strong rhythmic beat. Poor Mr. Bear's heart, on the other hand, is bluish in color, large, and round. If you look closely, you may notice that every beat seems to be a supreme struggle." He walked to the electrocardiographs and pushed a button on each one, freezing the images on the screens. Pointing to Wile E's E.C.G., he said, "Look familiar? Normal P-wave followed by a tight QRS complex and finishing on time with a normal T-wave. Each cycle nice and uniform. Are we agreed?" he asked, looking at us. "Now, let's look at Mr. Bear's E.C.G. Someone tell me what you see."

Ellen Green raised her hand. "He's missing QRS waves," she said. "I see three P-waves and only one QRS."

"Excellent. What do you suppose is going on?" he asked.

"A weakened heart muscle stretches," Ellen said. "That can interfere with nerve conduction."

"I'll buy that. Any other ideas?"

As expected, David Cartwright, who always sat in the front row, was first to raise his hand. Around school, Cartwright was a type known as a "gunner", a student who typically spent more time studying than sleeping, eating, and playing combined. I had told Katy about him.

Katy had replied, "At the end of this long, hard road you've chosen, when you walk across that stage, your pockets full of Bs and Cs behind Cartwright and his pockets full of As, remember, everybody's diploma will read the same—Doctor."

"Yes, Mr. Cartwright," Dr. Clark said.

"I'd like to know something, sir. Is Bear on digitalis?"

"Why do you ask?" Dr. Clark said while suppressing a smirk.

"Because, Bear has a second-degree AV block. It's a classic symptom of digitalis toxicity."

Dr. Clark smiled. "Very impressive, Mr. Cartwright. It seems that Bear's owner became desperate this weekend when his condition significantly deteriorated. She doubled up on his digitalis dose."

Ronny leaned over and whispered in my ear, "That Cartwright is a pretty smart guy." I tried to answer him, but suddenly, I didn't feel well. The room was hot and staring at those beating hearts was nauseating.

The next half hour consisted of a series of experiments designed to create arrhythmias, abnormal heart beats. Wile E's oxygen flow was reduced by seventy-five percent. Bear was given an intravenous injection of Potassium. The effects on both E.C.G. recordings were discussed. I closed my eyes and repeated to myself, relax . . . breathe deeply . . . relax. Hard as I tried, I couldn't suppress the dizziness. I was breathing faster and faster.

"Before we send these great guys to their final resting place," Dr. Clark said, "let's look at the ultimate arrhythmia. It's called ventricular fibrillation, or as the boys in blue are fond of calling it, v-fib. A heart in v-fib will beat no more unless you just happen to be carrying a defibrillator in your back pocket."

He put on thick rubber gloves and signaled to both technicians to step back. He picked up a live electrical cord, the tips of the wires exposed, and touched the wires to Wile E's heart. Instantly, the rhythmic wave of his E.C.G. disappeared and was replaced by an erratic oscillation on the screen. His heart stopped beating, but quivered like Jell-O in a deep bowl.

I felt sweat running down my forehead to the bridge of my nose and drip off my chin. I could see Dr. Clark's lips moving, but I couldn't hear the words. I rested my head against the wall and felt myself begin to slump toward Ronny. The room turned gray and then faded into black.

I'm not sure how long I was unconscious. I began to regain my senses. I was comfortable, my head rested on what felt like a soft pillow. It was cradled by somebody's neck and shoulder—Ronny's.

Oh, my God, I thought as I struggled to sit up straight. I had passed out! My eyes were closed, but I sensed everyone looking at me. I heard voices, but couldn't make out what they were saying. I imagined they were talking about me.

"Did you see Humphreys? He fainted."

"What a wimp."

"Who the hell let him into this pool, anyway?"

I opened my eyes slowly and scanned the room. Nobody was looking at me. Dr. Clark was the only person talking. Everyone else was feverishly writing notes on their pads. They didn't see me! I can't believe it. I might be in the clear! Nobody knew I had fainted . . . except for Ronny. He must have been shocked initially, possibly questioned my intentions and yet, he didn't move. He sat still with my head on his shoulder for what must have seemed an eternity. Was he still in shock, or just buying time until after class when he could announce to the world, what an ass I was? I wondered if he had a price for his silence.

I turned to look at him. He was also writing notes on his pad. Without looking at me, he whispered, "Don't worry, Jim. Your secret is safe with me."

That evening, Katy met me as I came through the front door. "Well, how was your day?"

"It was great. Really great."

"Really? Tell me about it."

"I made a friend today," I said and smiled. "A very good friend . . . with a big heart." I put my arms around her. "Let's go take your clothes off and hunt for ticks."

MY FRIENDS WALK BAREFOOT

Chapter 3

A TALE OF TWO DUMMIES

Dr. Bill Romane had more clout than any other member of the entire faculty at the veterinary school. He had served as department head of the large animal hospital of the College of Veterinary Medicine at Texas A&M University for years until health problems forced him to give up the stress of administrative duties and move to the ranks of instructor. Having accepted his demotion must have been difficult for him, but it was a blessing for the students. He was a quiet man, but a passionate and demanding professor who challenged his students and asked them to put aside the textbooks and trust their senses.

Katy had finished her MS degree, accepted a job in southeastern New Mexico, and had moved several months ahead of me. Our final year consisted of classwork as well as 5-week clinical rotations, alternating from small animal to large animal, medicine to surgery. My last rotation was Equine Medicine. Twenty of us were assigned to be under the supervision of Dr. Romane.

We gathered in a treatment room around this icon of horse doctors. "Ladies and gentlemen," he said in a soft voice, "let's go to work." We followed him into the horse barn, where over the next two hours, each of us was assigned the cases we were personally responsible for treating.

I was assigned four patients, a sorrel quarter horse mare with a bad wound on a front leg that required daily antibiotics and bandage changes, a bay gelding with pulmonary disease requiring twice-a-day antibiotics and nebulizer breathing treatments, and a young colt with generalized dermatitis that required daily antibiotics and a medicated bath every other day. The last case to be assigned was a two-year-old Arabian stallion that had been kicked in the scrotum by another horse.

"Humphreys," Dr. Romane said. "This one is yours."

"What am I supposed to do with this idiot, Doc?" I asked. "Massage his balls?"

I immediately regretted my careless sarcasm. For a few seconds, Dr. Romane stood motionless. Then he slowly removed his glasses, took a handkerchief from his pocket, wiped the lenses, and put them back on. "For ten to fifteen minutes, three times a day," he said without looking at me. "Class dismissed." He walked away.

Who's the idiot now, I thought. "I sure hope he was kidding," I said to no one in particular, but the guy standing next to me laughed.

"I wouldn't bet on it, Jim. Good luck, man."

We had five minutes to get to our first class. I had no time to worry about it now. The afternoon was long, classrooms were hot, and Applied Neurology—the last class of the day—was murder. By the end of the day, I was ready to go home, but then I remembered I still had horses to treat. I gathered my notes and textbook, put them in my backpack, and headed out to the horse barn. Rounding the first corner, I ran into a crowd, mostly students and a group of very distinguished professors including Dr. Romane. They hovered around a single stall. "What's going on?" I asked.

Rusty Marley answered. He was one of my classmates. "The *dummy foal* just arrived."

"The what?" I asked.

"The *dummy foal* everybody's been talking about. He just got here from Houston. Where the hell have you been?"

"What's a *dummy foal*?"

He looked at me and shook his head. "Apparently, the mare had a hard time delivering this baby. I guess he was deprived of oxygen for a while. He was born pretty well brain dead. He can't stand, can't see, can't suck. When a baby is so bad that he can't even suck, he's called a dummy foal."

"Why don't they put him down?" I asked, expressing what I thought was an obvious question.

Rusty pointed to a tall, bald man standing in the center of the ring of professors waving his hands and barking orders to everyone.

"See that guy? He's the owner. I guess he paid an ungodly amount of money to get his mare bred."

"Who is he?" I asked.

"Some hotshot neurosurgeon from Houston," Rusty said. "I hear he's not very nice. Apparently, he thinks he knows more than any of our professors about what's best for this baby. He told Dr. Romane he doesn't want any students messing with his colt. Dr. Carter's in charge. Don't think he's very thrilled about it."

Kent Carter, a graduate of Colorado State University, was a husky man with thin hair and a bushy mustache. He was confident, but nice and easy going, unlike some first-year residents who enjoyed treating students like lower class citizens. He was truly brilliant and yet, he always considered us colleagues rather than students.

Dr. Romane, who had been kneeling next to the non-responsive foal, stood up. "Okay, people, I suggest you all get your cases treated and get home," he ordered.

The crowd began to disperse and I turned to Rusty. "So, I guess that little foal is worth a ton of money, huh?"

Dr. Carter walked past me and apparently heard my question. He looked over his shoulder at his new patient. "He's not worth a plug nickel now."

I had an apology to make and waited for the crowd to leave. "Uh, Dr. Romane? About my stallion with the swollen testicles, sir . . ." I stopped and hoped he might overlook my previous stupid remarks.

"Just make sure he gets some exercise, Jim. Ten minutes of gentle walking and five ccs of Lasix, IM twice a day should do the trick," he said with a smile.

"Yes, sir," I said, relieved beyond words. It took me an hour and a half to finish my treatments. At last, I could go home.

The next morning, I walked into the horse barn and saw Dr. Carter with a couple of assistants as they worked on the brainless baby. The colt lay on an air mattress to prevent pressure sores. An intravenous line dripped life-sustaining fluid into his jugular vein. Dr. Carter removed a tube that he had passed through the colt's nose and into his stomach to deliver milk formula. That meant the foal still couldn't suck.

"How's he doing, Doc?" I asked.

"Not well at all," he answered. He didn't look up.

"You think he's gonna make it?"

"Nope."

"What does the owner have to say about him?" I asked, but suddenly felt I had overstepped my bounds.

This time, Dr. Carter looked up at me. I saw the contempt in his eyes.

"The owner's an asshole," he said. Then he lowered his voice, placed a gentle hand on his patient, and sighed. "But that's not this little guy's fault, so we'll do what we can to help him."

I responded with a nod, said nothing, and left. I finished treatments with ten minutes to spare before class. Ahead of me was another day of ninety degrees with ninety-five percent humidity.

The last afternoon class of every Tuesday was a grand rounds session with Dr. Romane as our moderator. He randomly called on students to present their case to the class while he sat back and listened. The session was completely open to questions, constructive criticism, and advice from any student on any presented case. Dr. Romane occasionally interjected with, "Comments or questions?" but nothing else. He was very careful not to break his own rule. This was students' time.

After the final student presented her case, Dr. Romane announced, "Before I let you go, I've asked Dr. Carter to present a particularly difficult case to you."

Dr. Carter gave a synopsis of the dummy foal. He articulated his patient's problems professionally. He followed with a review of his plan of action and progress report. He shook his head. "On top of all his other problems, the colt has developed pneumonia. Any questions?" he asked with a deep sigh. "If not, I'd better get back to him." He sounded tired and discouraged. He left the room. I felt sorry for him.

Charlie Copenhaver, one of the less shy members of our class, asked, "Dr. Romane, who is this guy who owns the baby?"

"His name is Theodore Clinton . . . the III. He comes from a long line of very prestigious doctors. All surgeons. All Texas A&M grads. I've known his grandfather for years. Nice guy."

"So, what's with this guy?" Charlie asked. "Surely, he must know this baby's not going to make it. Why doesn't he just put him to sleep?"

Dr. Romane sighed. "He's an asshole, Charlie." The room went silent. Dr. Romane had never used that language. "Good session, everyone," he continued. "Get to your cases and get home."

The following day was uneventful. It was six in the evening. I was in the treatment room changing the bandage on my sorrel mare's leg wound when Dr. Romane walked in.

"How's she looking, Jim?" he asked as he peeked over my shoulder.

3 – A Tale of Two Dummies

"Looking good, Doc." I buttered a gauze sponge with antibiotic cream, placed it over the wound, and began applying a new bandage.

"When do you want to send her home?" he asked.

"Probably next week. The wound is contracting well, but it needs more time."

"I agree," he said. "How are your other cases doing?"

"Well, my dermatitis case is almost cleared up, no more scabs or new pustules. I'm thinking he should be able to go home Monday or Tuesday of next week," I said. "My gelding's breathing is much better. He still has a cough, but it's less frequent and less intense, and the stallion is looking great. His scrotum is back to normal size. The little shit's gettin' to be a pain in the butt when I give him his injections," I chuckled. "He's feeling much better."

Dr. Romane seemed satisfied. "Okay. Stop the Lasix and give me an update tomorrow. I'll try to get him out of here on Friday. That'll be one less case you have to worry about. Good job, Bud."

"Thanks, Dr. Romane," I said as I finished applying the bandage. Another twelve-hour day for the record books.

That evening, I ate a TV dinner and watched a television sitcom that required neither close attention nor interpretive skills. At times like this, I really missed Katy. I was about ready for bed when I suddenly remembered—I have night duty tomorrow!

Night duty was one of the least desirable services required of all senior students. In the large animal hospital, night duty was shared by two students, one from medicine and one from surgery rotation. An easy night might mean two or three ten o'clock treatments followed by a decent night's sleep whereas, critical patients requiring lots of care could make for a long night.

The following morning, I threw a change of underwear and socks, a toothbrush, and a chocolate bar into my backpack. There would be no time to come home after class. I was delighted to find out that my good friend Ronny Hooker was assigned to be my partner for night duty. He was on the Equine Surgery rotation and we hadn't seen each other for a good while. I looked forward to some time for the two of us to catch up.

That evening, I finished treating my horses with an hour to spare before reporting for duty and headed to the school cafeteria. It was empty except for a few professors drinking coffee, and there was Ronny, seated alone and eating a sandwich. "Jim." He waved to get my attention.

I grabbed a sandwich and a soda. "Good to see you, Ronny. Looks like it's you and me tonight."

"Just like old times."

"How's surgery going?" I asked.

"It's been great. Dr. Auer put a mare's shattered carpus back together today. The guy's a genius. How are things in medicine?"

I told him about the stallion with the swollen testicles. We both laughed when I elaborated about my comments to Dr. Romane. We had just begun to enjoy each other's company when we realized it was time to report for duty.

Dr. Carter sat at a desk as he finished his medical records. We approached him. "Hey, Doc," I said. "Long day, huh?"

"Yeah," he said, and rubbed his temples with the tips of his fingers. "You guys ready?"

"Yes, sir," we answered simultaneously.

"Okay. What's going on in surgery, Ronny?"

"There's not much, Doc," Ronny answered. "Dr. Auer asked me to check on his case sometime tonight. Everybody else should be good till tomorrow."

"Sounds good. I wish I could be that easy on you guys, but I need you to get temps on the dun mare in stall fifty-three and the colt in seventy-one sometime between nine and midnight. I'm not expecting a problem, but if either of them is running a fever, call me, okay? And then, there's the dummy foal. Jim knows all about him, Ronny. I'm sorry you guys, but I really need a record of his vitals every three hours. That means nine o'clock, twelve, three, and six. The owner is driving up from Houston tonight after work. We can count on him being here first thing in the morning and I want to be able to show him that we've been on top of everything."

"Don't worry about a thing," Ronny said. "We'll take care of him."

Dr. Carter smiled for the first time in a while. "Thanks, guys."

"Get some sleep, Doc," I said. "We've got it covered."

Ronny looked at me as Dr. Carter slowly walked out the door. "He doesn't look so good."

"He's worn out," I said, then proceeded to give him details on the dummy foal.

"Doesn't sound like this colt has much of a chance," Ronny said. "Why doesn't the owner put him down?"

"That's the million-dollar question, Ronny. I hear he's a real jerk."

"Well, we have a couple of hours before first treatments," Ronny said. "Let's go check out the sleeping quarters. I hear they finally put a microwave in there."

The night duty receptionist sat at her desk to take in-coming emergency calls. Our room was directly across the hall from her desk. It was a small room with two single beds, a bathroom, refrigerator, television and yes, a microwave oven.

We sat on our beds and visited for a while, then watched TV until it was time for the nine o'clock check. Our first stop was Ronny's surgery patient. Next, we checked temperatures on the two horses in stalls fifty-three and seventy-one. Finally, we checked on the foal. While I took his temperature, Ronny recorded his heart and respiratory rates, then listened to his lungs with his stethoscope.

"He sounds a bit raspy, Jim," he said with concern.

"He's been that way since yesterday afternoon," I said. "Dr. Carter added some antibiotic to his IV fluids last night. He's had 500 ccs since the last check. Just what the schedule calls for."

Ronny ran his hand gently down the colt's neck and across his chest. "He's completely unresponsive," he said. "This is so unfair to this little guy."

"I agree. Everybody agrees, except the owner."

The medical chart hung on the stall gate. We recorded everything, including comments about the harsh lung sounds. We initialed the chart and hung it back on the gate.

3 – A Tale of Two Dummies

Ronny took a final look at the foal and shook his head. "Unbelievable. Let's get to bed." We set an alarm for twelve o'clock and turned the light out.

I was sound asleep when I heard someone bang on the door. We both fumbled out of our beds and as I stumbled in the dark to look for the light switch, the door flew open, the light came on, and a tall, bald man stood and stared at us.

"What in the hell are you idiots doing in here fast asleep while my colt is out there dying?" My eyes struggled to adjust to the light while the man raged, "You have two minutes to get dressed and get your asses out there!" He slammed the door on his way out.

"Who the hell was that?" Ronny asked, still half asleep.

"I'm not sure, but I think he's the owner of the colt."

"What the hell is he doing here? How did he get past the receptionist?"

"Hell if I know. We better get out there." I looked at the alarm clock. It was ten minutes till twelve. We threw on coveralls and boots and ran out the door.

Dr. Theodore Clinton . . . the III waited for us at the stall while he paced back and forth with hands on his hips. If he'd had a gun, I believe he would have shot both of us.

"Well, don't just stand there you idiots. Check this colt out, now!"

He snatched the medical record off the gate. Ronny and I knelt next to the colt. Ronny pulled his stethoscope from his pocket and listened to the colt's heart and lungs while I checked his temperature and the color of his gums. The IV fluids ran according to schedule, his heart and respiratory rates remained stable. His temperature read normal and his color was good.

I was mad. This guy was outta line! I took a deep breath and tried to stay calm. "What made you think he was dying, sir?"

"Easy, Jim," Ronny whispered.

Dr. Teddy stared at me with cold, black eyes. "Shut up!" he barked. "I'm the one asking the questions here!" He was definitely intimidating, but I was done listening to him. I glanced at Ronny who shook his head, very subtly. I read his lips. "Don't do it, Jim. Please don't do it," he whispered.

And then, good sense gave way to bad judgment. I stood firm, erect, set my shoulders, and pointed my finger at Dr. Clinton. "I don't know who the hell you think you are, mister, but we're not going to put up with your crap anymore."

Ronny stood frozen.

The man looked at me, incredulously with narrowed eyes. "What did you say?"

My heart beat faster and I felt sweat dripping down my forehead. "Dr. Carter gave us very specific instructions and we have followed them to the letter, sir. If you'll pass me the medical record, I'll update it and you'll see that there has been absolutely no change in this colt's condition all night. His vitals are stable."

"Do you have any idea who you're talking to?" Dr. Clinton said and slammed the record to the ground. "I'll have your head handed to you on a stick for this, you stupid kid."

3 – A Tale of Two Dummies

Oh well, I thought. Too late to turn back now. "You have one of two choices, mister. You can walk out that door, get in your car, and leave or I'll call security and have them drag your ass out in handcuffs." My mouth was so dry that those last words almost didn't make it past my lips.

His hands shook as they searched for something to grasp. His mouth was open and his lips quivered like Jell-O. "You're going to pay for this," he said. "Whether my colt lives or dies, I'll see that you never graduate." He turned around and walked out of the barn.

"Holy shit, Jim," Ronny said.

"Yeah, I know," I replied. "Me and my big mouth. What was I thinking, Ronny?" I sighed. "Don't worry, man. This one is all on me."

When we got back to our room, I said, "Don't set the alarm, Ronny. I won't be sleeping tonight anyway." He didn't argue. As I lay in bed in the dark, my mind repeated over and over, you really screwed up this time, Humphreys. Who's the dummy now?

At three o'clock, I went out to the barn. The baby's condition had not changed. I took his vitals and recorded them. God, I hope that man doesn't show up again.

I wandered up and down the halls for the next hour and wondered if this was the end of the road for me. I had threatened a client. Just how powerful was Dr. Clinton? Did he have the means to keep me from graduating? All the years of hard work, the sleepless nights, stress beyond definition, dreams of someday becoming a veterinarian—was it all for naught? I finished treating my own cases in time to make the six o'clock check on the foal and returned to the night room.

Ronny was dressed. "Did you get any sleep?" he asked as he brushed his teeth.

"Naw. I checked on the colt at three and just now. There's no change. Listen," I said. "I'm gonna get out of here and go home for a bit before class. Might as well get cleaned up before I face the firing squad."

"Hey, we're in this together, Jim. Don't you worry," he said. "I'll back you up." He checked his watch. "Guess I'd better get to studying. I have a test this morning." He saw the worried look on my face. "It's gonna be okay, Jim. By the way, thanks for letting me sleep."

I had never felt so tired and scared as I did when I walked into my first class that morning. I didn't hear a word of the lecture, but I did notice a young lady who walked across the room to Dr. Morris and whispered in his ear as he finished his summation.

"Class dismissed," he said. His eyes searched the crowd until he found me. "Humphreys! Dr. Boyd would like to see you in his office right away." Every eye in the room was on me as we filed out into the hallway.

Dr. Boyd was department head of the large animal hospital. It was a long walk to his office. My hands trembled as I knocked on his door and heard that authoritative voice.

"Come in."

I opened the door and walked in. He looked over the top of his glasses at me.

3 – A Tale of Two Dummies

"Come in and sit down, Jim."

I sat down as ordered. He removed his glasses and set them on his desk. We both remained silent for a moment. A wide smile spread across his face. "You really busted open a hornets' nest last night, young man."

I felt the tears well in my eyes. "I'm sorry, Dr. Boyd. I don't know what to say. The guy was a real jerk, sir."

He studied my face, as if trying to decide whether he saw any remorse. "Well, I think we're going to be okay," he chuckled. "Our receptionist was peeking around the corner and witnessed the whole thing. Sounds like you stared the devil in the eye . . . and he blinked."

I said nothing.

"Dr. Clinton assures me that he is going straight to Dean Shelton with his complaint," he said. "Luckily, Dean Shelton knows all about the great Dr. Clinton. I suspect nothing will come of this, but I want you to keep a low profile from now until graduation. Are we clear?" he asked with a stern look.

"Yes sir," I said. I stood and shook his hand. "Thanks, Dr. Boyd."

I felt overwhelmingly relieved as I walked down the hallway. Just maybe, I would survive this ordeal after all. I began to feel good about myself again and then I saw Dr. Romane walk in my direction. I prepared myself for the reprimand of my life. "Good morning, Dr. Romane."

He looked at me and shook his head. "Remind me never to piss you off."

I wasn't sure how to respond. "That's not funny, Doc. I've just spent the last ten hours wondering whether my career was down the toilet. I'm sorry, sir. What's gonna happen?"

"What's going to happen? Oh, I suspect, nothing. Dr. Clinton is loading up his foal as we speak and taking him to Don Levins' Equine Center in Houston. Why he didn't go there in the first place, I don't know. We tried our best, but he's not our problem anymore. I think Dr. Carter owes you a steak dinner," he chuckled. He put his hand on my shoulder. "You're going to be a good veterinarian, Jim. Just learn to keep that mouth of yours in check and you'll be all right." He patted me on the arm and walked past me. "How're your cases doing?" he asked.

"Doing well sir, doing well."

Monday morning arrived and I felt like a new man. Dr. Romane had sent the Arab stallion home on Friday. My respiratory and dermatitis cases were both ready to go home as well. I was changing the bandage on the sorrel mare when he came into the treatment room.

"Good morning, Dr. Romane," I said with a burst of enthusiasm. "I think she can go home this week."

He looked closely at the wound. "Yup. Maybe tomorrow. By the way, I heard something today you might be interested in."

"Oh yeah? What's that?"

"I got a call from Don Levins in Houston. It seems that Clinton showed up with his foal on Friday afternoon, yelling and screaming at everyone. Don took one look at the colt and gave Clinton two options—take his colt somewhere else or put him down. The old bird finally gave it up. Don put the foal to sleep. That baby is finally at peace."

He sighed. "This was a tough case, Jim . . . and a good lesson. You'll have a few more like this to deal with before you get to be my age." I turned and saw the face of an experienced, caring, wise teacher. "Never forget," he said. "Your duty is to your patient. Sometimes, that has to be in spite of your client." He paused and then, "But always, always, be what you are—professional."

I nodded and said, not a word.

"Well," he said. "You're about to run out of cases. Ready for some new ones?"

"You betcha, Doc. I'm ready for anything."

He smiled. "Yes sir . . . I believe you are."

MY FRIENDS WALK BAREFOOT

Chapter 4

A LESSON FROM SCRUTCH

We all called him "Scrutch," but not to his face. It wasn't meant to be disrespectful, but rather a name of endearment, a name that carried with it, the deepest respect that we held for him. He was like a father to us.

Dr. Leon Scrutchfield was forty years old and bore a stocky body on a five-foot-ten frame. His big round face sported a shiny complexion, a full red beard, and hair that showed signs of thinning. Scrutch was easy to spot in the hallway with his baggy pants and suspenders. He was undoubtedly a southerner, a graduate of the University of Missouri who spoke with a drawl and used terms like "Damn straight" and "Oh ma-gosh."

Scrutch had a successful private practice for many years. He gave that up to pursue a life-long dream—to teach. He came to Texas A&M and became a die-hard Aggie.

Lots of great professors came to A&M from all over the world. They were bright men and women, some leaders in their respective fields, exceptionally gifted individuals with published research papers and huge grants to back up their brilliance. Yet, if ever asked to pick a single teacher who was most influential with his students, many of us agreed it was Scrutch.

I always felt that Scrutch was one smart dude who had a burning passion and determination to make sure that no student of his would ever leave Texas A&M without also being one smart dude.

Passionate as he was about teaching, he occasionally loosened up, meeting with us on Friday afternoon at the Dixie Chicken for a beer. These were special times. The conversation ranged from the weather to the upcoming football game to the jazz festival to be held the coming weekend, but never . . . about school.

Graduation was a little over a month away. Soon, we would hold the coveted title that would precede our names—Doctor. The thought of it seemed a bit pretentious to me, but it was fun to brag among ourselves.

Once a year, Dr. Scrutchfield offered an elective course in Equine Internal Medicine, a four-week comprehensive and intensive course. For anyone wanting to be a horse doctor, this course was invaluable and yet, after years of lectures, long days, and late nights studying for exams, our brains were fried. We were anxious to get out into the real world. Of the 120 students still left in my class, only fifteen signed up—including my good friend Ronny Hooker and me.

It was Monday of our last week of school. Scrutch's class had lived up to its reputation, so much information and so little time. We walked into the room as he wrote on the blackboard. It was large and when he was done, the board was filled with line after line of information that at the time, seemed incomprehensible.

4 – A Lesson from Scrutch

"Good morning, kids," Dr. Scrutchfield said. He liked to refer to us as his kids. "You've all done a remarkable job of cramming a whole lot of stuff into your brains these past few weeks. I'm proud of you," he said. "Today, I thought we might do something a little different. Instead of me telling you what's going on, you're going to tell me what's going on." He pointed to the board behind him. "I've listed four cases. Each of these horses was presented to our hospital by referring veterinarians. As you can see, each case has a list of clinical signs of disease. The information I'm giving you is sketchy and may not be enough for a definitive diagnosis. The point is, I want you to *think!* Study each one carefully and come up with a differential. I want your first, second, and third most likely reasons for each horse's clinical signs," he instructed. "This is a class exercise, so team up and get to work. I'll go get some coffee and be back in thirty minutes. Oh, yeah, remember . . . *Think outside the box."*

Ellen Green, one of the more out-spoken members of our class and a natural leader, stood and said, to no one's surprise, "Okay, everyone. I suggest we move our desks into a large circle facing each other." We all agreed and did as Ellen suggested. "Let's see," she continued. "Case number one is a two-year-old bay gelding stumbling on all four feet. Acute onset of symptoms, his vitals are normal, he has a good appetite, he has free range of a ten-acre pasture, and that's it. Sounds like he just can't walk a straight line. Ideas, anyone?"

Ronny Hooker spoke up. "I think he's off neurologically. Could be a spinal problem. All four legs are involved, so probably cervical. How about *Wobbler Syndrome?"* He referred to an illness which describes a horse with instability in the cervical spine. Laxity between two adjacent vertebrae in the neck allows the spinal cord to be pinched resulting in loss of feeling in all four legs.

"Good choice, Ronny. I like it. Are we in agreement?" Ellen asked. Everyone nodded.

I thought of another possibility. "It could be vestibular disease. Maybe a guttural pouch infection that spread to the middle and inner ear causing loss of balance," I said. Most of my classmates agreed, others remained silent.

Another classmate suggested *Equine Herpes Virus* which often affects the spinal cord. Two more possibilities were presented and after some discussion, we selected our top three choices and Ellen recorded them on a piece of paper.

Case number two was a five-year-old grey mare that was found at morning feeding with her eyes closed and head pressed tightly against a corner of her stall. She moaned, was non-responsive to her owner's voice, and was unable to eat or drink. Western and Eastern *Equine Encephalomyelitis*, both mosquito-borne viral diseases not uncommon to the area were obvious choices. A more extensive list of possibilities was compiled and again, we picked our top three most likely diagnoses.

Our third case was a yearling Arabian colt that had suddenly gone blind. He was confined to a stall made of steel pipe recently painted by a rancher whose tack room was full of old paint. It was likely that a young, energetic colt licked the pipes. That's what horses do when they are bored. Lead poisoning immediately rose to the top of the list.

4 – A Lesson from Scrutch

I noticed the excitement on the faces of this circle of young, soon-to-be doctors. I felt the same. Energized by the task that Scrutch had given us, we discussed, we argued, we challenged each other to defend our diagnoses, but ultimately, we arrived at agreement on the probable etiologies. All the years of sleepless nights, the endless studying, the stress-induced heart arrhythmias, and duodenal ulcers came down to this, a chance to lay it all out on the table. It was well worth the price we had paid. No one leaves here today without being one smart dude, I thought.

We had started a discussion of our fourth case when Scrutch walked into the room with his Texas Aggie mug full of coffee in one hand and a half-eaten doughnut in the other. "How we doin', kids?" he asked.

"Almost done, Dr. Scrutchfield," Ellen answered. All of us agreed that cases one, two, and three were neurologically abnormal. We also agreed that case number four was different. This was a fifteen-year-old sorrel mare that seemed to have problems swallowing and periodic episodes of violent head shaking. She coughed, gagged, and dunked her nose into her water trough. She pawed at the side of the trough, frustrated by her apparent inability to drink the water she desperately wanted and needed.

"I think I know this one," Ellen said, barely able to contain her excitement. "I saw a case just like this last month. This horse has *choke*."

"Choke" refers to an esophageal obstruction which typically occurs when a horse swallows a bolus of food that's too dry. The food makes it halfway down the esophagus toward the stomach and gets stuck. It's extremely painful. This was consistent with symptoms shown by case number four.

I had never seen a case of choke and I could tell by the confused looks on the faces of my classmates, they had never seen one either. Because Ellen seemed very sure of herself, we all agreed.

Then suddenly, a quiet voice we hadn't heard from yet, spoke up. "Back home, we had cows eat a mesquite branch on occasion, said Mark Miller. He was a shy member of our class. "It generally gets hung up at the back of their tongue," he continued. "They act a lot like this. Don't think I've ever seen a horse do the same thing, but it's possible."

"I agree with Mark," I said. "Whether mesquite or something else, we sure need to consider a foreign body." Everyone nodded in agreement and Ellen wrote it down. A few other possibilities were discussed including *vesicular stomatitis*, a viral infection similar to hoof and mouth disease which caused painful oral ulcers.

"We're ready, Dr. Scrutchfield," Ellen said after we had picked our top three diagnoses.

"Show me what you got, Ellen," Dr. Scrutchfield said as he took a bite of his doughnut.

Ellen passed the list around the circle. It was beautifully constructed in perfect outline form with each case written in bold print and the diagnoses listed neatly, one below the other. Scrutch took it, sat at his chair, put his feet up on his desk, and studied it.

4 – A Lesson from Scrutch

I kept my eyes fixed on Scrutch while the rest of the class relaxed and whispered to each other. His face was expressionless for a long time. He began running his fingers through his hair and scratching his beard. He took deep breaths along with an occasional but subtle shake of his head. Something wasn't right. He seemed frustrated, disgusted, or both.

Finally, he placed his glasses on his desk, sat up straight, and rubbed his eyes. "Okay, people," he said. "I want everybody to turn around and look at me."

People? We had just been demoted from his kids to people. Something was wrong. Now, with more fear than anticipation, we rearranged our desks and sat down.

He held our list high above his head. "Before we start," he said, "does anyone have anything to add to this list?"

There was no answer.

"Anyone at all?"

There was still no answer.

He sighed. "Okay, next question. Do we see any common denominator in these four cases?"

"We all agreed that the first three seem to be neurological," Ellen said. "Case four is the exception . . . we think."

Scrutch nodded. "Okay. Let's go over this." Instead of reading the list chronologically, he selected our diagnoses randomly. "Encephalomyelitis, Vesicular Stomatitis, Wobbler. Very good. I like them." He paused and chuckled. "Lead poisoning! I wondered if you would take the bait on that one."

Everybody smiled, except for Scrutch. "You did a good job," he said. "Your answers are right on target." He sighed and shook his head. "Do you remember the last thing I said before I left the room? *'Think outside the box!'* Do you remember that? It's the one thing you didn't do. I'm sorry that I haven't done a better job of teaching you that and it saddens me."

The mood had changed. A minute ago, we were hot stuff. Now, we struggled to figure out what we had done wrong. Dr. Scrutchfield put the list on his desk and tapped it with the tips of his fingers. "You missed it, people. You missed it. All four of these horses had the same problem and it's nowhere to be found on this piece of paper."

He put his elbows on his desk, rested his chin on clinched fists, and closed his eyes. "I'm imagining you treating these horses. Let's take the first three since we all agree they're neurological. You're going to check their vitals, right? You're going to lift their upper lips and check the color of their gums. Then you'll get right next to them with your ophthalmoscopes and examine the retinas in both eyes, right?"

Nobody answered.

He continued, "All three of these horses will die, but not before they've put each one of you in mortal danger."

I felt cold. What in the world had we missed?

"Now, let's look at number four," Scrutch continued with his eyes still closed. "You're gonna have to pass a stomach tube to see if she has an esophageal impaction. If she's not a choke case, she's got something wrong in her mouth. That's what you decided, right?"

Again, nobody responded.

"So, you're gonna put a speculum in her mouth and take a look with your flashlight. When you don't see anything, you're gonna reach your hand way back in there and feel around for something, right?"

This time, he didn't wait for an answer. "Guess what, people. Number four is gonna die too and she just might take you with her!"

There was silence. My heart pounded and I could feel the arteries in my neck pulsate.

"You see, she is also a neurological case," he continued. "The muscles of her tongue and larynx that she needs to be able to swallow are paralyzed." He stopped . . . and opened his eyes.

I felt the tingling of goose bumps running up both of my arms. Oh my God. I get it! How could I have been so stupid? I scanned the room. Two or three of my classmates still looked completely confused, but the rest were like me, eyes and mouths wide open as if we had just witnessed a murder.

For the first time in a while, Scrutch smiled. He nodded, pleased to see that his kids finally saw the light. His eyes were caring, his voice, compassionate.

"Okay, kids. I want each of you to take a piece of paper and print your name at the top." We all did as our professor instructed.

"Now, I want you to address it to me. Write the following statement of promise, sign it, and pass it up front. Nobody gets out of here until I get all fifteen signed promises. If I find out, whether in ten, twenty, or thirty years from now, that one of you has broken that promise, I'll hunt you down and slap you in the face with your letter." He was serious. "Now, write—Dear Dr. Scrutchfield. I promise never to examine a sick horse without first taking a minute to consider the possibility of—Rabies."

*   *   *

It was twenty years before I saw Scrutch again. At a conference in San Antonio, Texas, a group of my classmates organized a reunion of the Class of 1981. True to his nature, Scrutch dropped in to say, "Hi." We talked for a long time and then I reminded him of that Monday morning twenty years earlier. "I gotta know, Dr. Scrutchfield, do you still have those fifteen letters?"

"Fifteen? Oh ma-gosh, Jim," he laughed. "I must have close to a thousand of those letters by now."

A smile spread across my face. Good ol' Scrutch. Still saving the lives of horses . . . and veterinarians.

Chapter 5
BUTTONS

In the fall of 1981, I was a young veterinarian, fresh out of school, full of ambition, enthusiasm, and just enough confidence to get in the way of common sense and good judgment. Buttons was a 14-year-old Boston terrier who had dedicated his entire life to the happiness of Geneva Williams, an 80-year-old widow without a single person in the world to claim as family, except Buttons.

Buttons was a typical Boston Terrier with a face that looked like he had run into the back of a parked car. His turned-up nose was complimented by a severe under-bite and large bug eyes, one brown, the other blue. The crooked nub of his tail shot back and forth from side to side with a distinct rhythm that seemed to keep perfect time with each breath that poured from his constricted nostrils. His dull, bristly hair, a sign of old age, was overshadowed only by the cold color of his tongue which closely matched his blue eye. Buttons had advanced congestive heart failure. The morning that we met was not one of his better days and I wasn't smart enough at the time to know that he was dying.

Our hospital receptionist, Polly, knew her all our patients well. She had stood guard at that desk for twenty-five years and every dog, cat, bird, or rabbit that came through the front door was her "kid". I studied the morning schedule when Mrs. Williams stepped into the office with Buttons. Polly realized immediately that he was in trouble. She slipped out of her desk and with the swiftness and grace of an eagle, she swooped down on Buttons, snatched him from his mother's arms and rushed past me, back to the emergency treatment area and delivered him into the capable hands of Tina, our technician, who immediately covered his face with a mask, started the flow of oxygen, and yelled, "Dr. T! I need you right now!"

Dr. T was a big man, six foot three, 220 pounds, with white hair and bushy eyebrows that hung on the tops of the thick glasses that accentuated the bags under his eyes. He was my boss.

Dr. T and I arrived at the treatment room at the same time. Tina handed him a stethoscope. Oxygen filtered its way deep into Buttons' lungs. His starved muscles relaxed and the distress in his eyes began to subside. His labored breathing eased and the color of his tongue returned to a more normal pink. Dr. T shifted his stethoscope back and forth, up and down over Button's chest. He listened with the intensity of someone defusing a bomb for what seemed, minutes. Finally satisfied with his evaluation, he handed the stethoscope to me.

"Give me your assessment and recommendation, young man." I placed one end of the stethoscope to my ears and the other end on Buttons' chest, expecting to hear the usual melody of a beating heart—lub-dub, lub-dub, lub-dub. It's a very simple two-beat, repeating sound

5 - Buttons

that continues over and over every day and night, year after year, all produced by this amazing little muscle that we all take for granted. The rhythm was not what I expected to hear, but rather a loud and rapid whoosh, whoosh, whoosh. There was no clarity to the heartbeat, as if he had swallowed a washing machine.

Like most dogs with congestive heart failure, Buttons' problem had started years earlier. It may have been a breed predisposition, a defect in his bloodline, or it may have been due to his "dirty mouth". Tartar on his teeth accumulated, accompanied by millions of colonies of bacteria which hid within the confines of his trashy mouth and caused his gums to recede, exposing the unprotected tooth roots. Opportunistic bacteria rushed into Button's blood stream, stuck to his heart valves, resulting in scar tissue.

Regardless of the reason, Buttons' heart valves were diseased and no longer opened easily or sealed tightly. Half of the blood pushed forward by each heartbeat, as if swimming in the ocean against the waves in high surf, escaped back through the damaged valves. The pressure within his heart increased, his heart muscle weakened and stretched. The nerves that governed the rhythm and rate of his heartbeat also stretched creating interruptions in nerve impulses. With a total disruption of the electrical system on which it depended as well as weakened muscles fibers incapable of proper contraction, a once-healthy heart now lived minute to minute.

Reluctantly, I looked up only to see Dr. T's furrowed eyebrows twitching with the impatience of a thoroughbred at the starting gate of the big race.

"Young man," he repeated, "give me your assessment and recommendation."

My mouth was dry, my tongue stuck to anything it touched. "He sounds pretty bad," I said. What a profound statement that was, I realized. I gathered all the courage I could muster, "but I think we can save him."

"Save him, huh? How do you expect to do that, young man?" Dr. T asked with an unpleasant facial expression that I had become accustomed to. He was fond of calling me "young man." I think it was his way of letting me know where I stood on the professional ladder, the top considered *the well-versed boss man* rung and the lowest, *the little more than ignorant* rung. My spot was somewhere between the ground and the first rung.

I really wanted to say, "It's amazing how far modern medicine has brought us from those dark ages when you guys were crawling out from under rocks, old geezer," but I remembered how my undisciplined mouth had gotten me in trouble in the past. I called on better judgement and said, "I have a plan."

Polly burst into the room. "Would somebody please come talk to this lady," she exclaimed through flared nostrils. "She's already left a lake of tears in my reception room and she is ready to put Buttons to sleep."

Dr. T looked at me with his patented sardonic grin. "Ok, hotshot, go present your plan to your client."

Geneva Williams sat on a bench as I walked into the reception area. Her grey hair was uncombed and she wore a heavy coat which covered undergarments and slippers. It was obvious she had left her house in a hurry. Her eyes were full of tears. Dark rings that colored her eyelids confirmed a sleepless night.

"Hi, Mrs. Williams. I'm Dr. Humphreys."

"How's my buddy?" she asked, her voice trembling.

"He's stable. We have him on oxygen. He's relaxing now."

"I knew this day had to come eventually, Dr. Humphreys," she said. "You know, it's just been the two of us since my husband died. I'm having a hard time giving him up, but I think he's ready and I need to *let him go.*"

The time had come for me to exert some authority, to put the knowledge I had worked so hard to gain, into action. I dove in headfirst. "I want to talk to you about that, Mrs. Williams. You see, I think we might be able to help Buttons. Maybe get him back on track." I wasn't sure I sounded very convincing, but it was a start.

The news took her by surprise. "Really," she said as she tried to control her excitement. "You mean you think you can fix my Buttons' heart?" Suddenly there was a hint of life back in her face. The tone of her voice changed from that of despair to one of hope.

For the next twenty minutes, I explained the intricacies of Buttons' problem and the plan that I had formulated to put life back into his damaged heart. We talked about *furosemide*, the diuretic that would force Buttons' kidneys to release more fluid lowering his blood pressure and relieving the stress on his heart. We talked about *digitalis*, the miracle drug that would slow his heart rate and increase the strength of each contraction, giving him a more efficient pump.

Our conversation switched to diet and controlled exercise. A smile spread across her face. Her tears had dried and there was excitement and enthusiasm in her voice. With a brand-new shot of confidence and a young and brilliant doctor by her side, she felt alive again.

At this very proud moment in my life, I noticed the door leading to the back hallway open ever so slightly. Although I couldn't see him, I heard Dr. T's voice.

"Dr. Humphreys, could I see you for a minute, please?" There was a hint of urgency in his voice, one that meant, *"Right now!"*

I gently placed my hand on Mrs. Williams' shoulder. "I'll be right back," I said.

By the look on Dr. T's face, I knew immediately that something was very wrong. I shut the door behind me and listened. As if in slow motion, my world began to unravel. "Buttons is dead," he said.

"What?"

"Buttons is dead," Dr. T repeated slowly, deliberately.

"He can't be! I just spent 20 minutes convincing Mrs. Williams that I could save her dog. He can't be dead." I felt cold.

Dr. T lowered his head, sighed, then looked at me. There was a hint of compassion that I had never seen in him before. "He's dead," he said.

It was a very low point in my life. I was at a complete loss. "What do I do now?" I asked.

He cleared his throat. "My suggestion is that you tell your client you were a little too late."

5 - Buttons

Too late? What kind of lame excuse is that, I thought. I started to sweat profusely and I felt nauseated.

"Do you need a little help with this?" Dr. T asked.

"No," I said, "I can handle it." Handle what, I wondered. I just got through telling this sweet lady that her dog was going to be fine and now I have to tell her that he's dead? Why didn't they teach us how to deal with this when we were in school? Maybe they did and I wasn't listening. What am I going to do?

I stepped back into the reception room where I found my client just as I had left her, still with a smile as though the whole world had been lifted off her shoulders. I can't do this to her, I thought. How will she handle the shock? I searched my mind frantically for the answer. I can't do this to her! Then it hit me. What if we went back to her original intentions of putting Buttons to sleep? Wouldn't that make it easier on her? It was bizarre and deceptive, but I just knew it was in Mrs. Williams' best interest. I'll take it slow and easy, let it be . . . her decision. Yes, that would be much easier on her. I had to ignore the fact that Buttons was dead and somehow convince her to put him to sleep.

I sat down next to this wonderful lady who had put her deepest trust in me and started down a path of no return. "There are a few potential complications we need to talk about, Mrs. Williams."

"What do you mean, Doctor?" she asked. I saw the look on her face change.

"I need to make sure you're going to be comfortable giving Buttons his medications—for the rest of his life. You'll be responsible for giving Buttons several pills twice a day."

"Oh my. Buttons doesn't take pills well," she said. I heard the tone of her voice change.

"Hmm, that could be a problem." I continued my case. "By the way, one of these medications could make him sick."

"Oh, my word, I wouldn't want that."

I could see her struggle with all the details of Buttons' treatment schedule, which I assured her, were essential to his survival. Whenever our conversation presented the opportunity, I introduced another complication that she had not counted on. She became less and less anxious to address a challenge that might give her some extra time with her beloved Buttons, but—at what cost to him? He was old and he had lived a wonderful life. Perhaps she owed it to him to let him go.

She looked at me and through tired, sad eyes said, "Dr. Humphreys, I really think maybe the best thing for Buttons is to put him to sleep."

I felt like I had just stolen from my own mother and yet, somehow, there was a feeling of supreme relief. "Perhaps you're right, Mrs. Williams. I completely understand and respect your decision."

She reached out and held my hand tightly. "Will you take care of this for me?"

"Of course I will, ma'am," I said. We sat in silence, hand in hand for several minutes and I began to relax. She took a Kleenex from her purse and wiped the tears from her eyes. Then came the dagger.

"Doctor, I'd like to see him one last time so I can say goodbye," she said with a sorrowful smile.

My heart dropped like a rock. How could this be happening? How could I not have seen this coming? Why hadn't I just told the truth! Time to think outside the box!

"I don't think that's a good idea, Mrs. Williams. I really don't think he'll even recognize you." That was definitely the understatement of my short career. "I think it would be best for both of you if you were to remember him when he was a happy boy." I had nothing left to say. I had resigned myself unconditionally to whatever was in the cards, and what I deserved.

The next few minutes drifted like hours. We sat together in complete silence. When she was ready, I helped her stand. She nodded and gave me a hug. "Thank you, Dr. Humphreys." She turned and walked out the door.

I glanced to my right and saw Polly, mouth wide open as her head shook from side to side. "Wow. How did you pull that one off?" she asked in complete shock.

"I don't feel so good," I said.

The rest of the day was little more than a blur. I walked down the hallway toward the treatment room where I was met by Dr. T's partner, Dr. Mike, also my employer who had been at a ranch fertility-testing bulls all day.

"I hear you had a bad day," he said.

"I don't even know what to say, Mike. It was awful. Did you hear the details?"

"Yup," he said with a grin that escalated to a laugh. "I've heard some real doozies, Jim, but yours takes the cake."

He realized I wasn't in the mood for humor. He walked up to me and threw his arm around my shoulders. "There are two things to remember about a mistake, Jim. Number one is that we all make them. Secondly, the smart guy learns a valuable lesson from the mistake and puts it behind him." He slapped me on the back and said as he walked away, "I think you're a smart guy." Those were words I really needed to hear just then. It was the beginning of a life-long brotherhood between Mike and me.

I walked in the front door of our cozy house. Katy met me with a tender kiss and a smile, generally the perfect ending to a long day.

She gazed into my eyes and her smile disappeared. She sighed deeply. "Uh oh," she said.

"You won't believe what happened to me today," I said as I shook my head.

"Why don't you tell me all about it."

And so I did, and with every sentence I spoke, I became increasingly embarrassed and upset. "I really did think I was doing what was best for her."

Katy cleared her throat. Then she chuckled and ended with her hands clasped over her mouth to contain her laughter. I didn't see it coming.

"This isn't supposed to be funny," I said. She reached for my hand.

"It's not funny, sweetheart. I'm sad for Mrs. Williams. Really, I am, but there wasn't anything else you could have done except . . .

5 - Buttons

maybe tell the truth? What I'm laughing about is the fact that I've known you since we were kids and I can't believe what a pickle you got yourself into. What in the world were you thinking?" She gave me a hug and suggested, "Why don't you go to bed early?"

"I think I will. Wake me if I sleep longer than next week."

Ten weeks later, Mrs. Williams walked through the front door of our office with her new puppy, a scrappy, eight-week-old Boston Terrier—Buttons II.

MY FRIENDS WALK BAREFOOT

Chapter 6
YELLOW MAGIC

Dr. Mike was a great boss. He had the admiration and respect of the entire staff. He had earned that distinction by his actions and the mutual respect that he showed for them. It was a true joy to work with this man. In contrast, Dr. T was an intimidating man. Those who worked for him quickly learned the importance of keeping busy, even if only in appearance, and to ask few questions of him. If he asked a question, the mandatory response was, "Yes sir" or "No sir" as if addressing a drill sergeant. Our receptionist, Polly, had nicknamed him Dr. Jekyll and Mr. Hyde. He was always the kind and compassionate Jekyll in the presence of a client, but the cruel and unfeeling Hyde to his hospital staff. It was an amazing transformation to witness.

Dr. T, Dr. Mike, and I shared the same office, a large rectangular room with a long narrow counter that seated three, with abundant bookshelves on the wall, a sofa, and an overstuffed chair. Mike was out of town for a few days on a pleasure trip. While Dr. T reviewed his morning schedule, Polly appeared at the door to our office.

"Mrs. Zimmerman is here to drop off Perky," she said. "She's going to Albuquerque for a few days and was hoping you had a minute to see her before she left." She hesitated for a moment and then, "I was thinking maybe you might introduce her to Dr. Humphreys." Dr. T stared at her without a hint of expression.

"Oh, you were, were you, thinking, that is? I'll be right there." Then he turned to me. "Have I ever told you about Mrs. Zimmerman, young man?"

"I don't believe so," I said.

"Her husband died unexpectedly about, oh, I guess it was ten years ago. She was in her late sixties at the time. Their kids were grown and gone leaving her pretty much on her own. One day, she was wandering through a pet store when she came upon a canary. She fell in love with him. He's been her faithful companion ever since. Don't know what she'd do without that little bird. Come on."

Dr. T and I walked into the reception room. Mrs. Zimmerman rose from the bench and threw her arms wide open with anticipation of a big hug.

"Doctor," she said with excitement. She was a lovely lady with white shoulder length hair, neatly brushed. Shiny skin covered her prominent cheek bones, her broad chin, and thin, bony hands. Her soft green eyes were magnified by the thick lenses of her glasses. She wore a bright yellow dress. Next to her on the bench was a birdcage holding a tiny canary, Perky.

"Good morning, young lady," Dr. T roared as he granted her the embrace she had so looked forward to. "You look more beautiful each time I see you."

6 – Yellow Magic

"Oh, Doctor," she said as she placed the palms of her hands on his cheeks. "You're incorrigible." They both laughed and then the tone of her voice changed. "I have to go to Albuquerque for a few days and I'm worried about Perky. His pretty yellow feathers don't seem as shiny as they should be and he hasn't been singing to me for the past week," she said. "Normally, I wouldn't dream of leaving him alone when he's not feeling well, but today is my grandson's birthday. My son and daughter in law are having a party for him tonight and I simply must be there. You know, I don't see well enough to drive anymore, but my neighbor is willing to drive me up and back."

"He's not going to be alone, darlin'. He's going to be with me," Dr. T said without so much as looking at the bird.

"I know he's getting old, Doc," she said. "I don't expect to be able to keep him forever. I just want him to be comfortable."

"Don't you worry about a thing," Dr. T said. "He's in good hands. There's nothing wrong with Perky that a little *yellow magic* won't take care of."

"Yellow magic?" she asked, with great curiosity.

"My little secret," he whispered, holding a forefinger to his lips. "Now, there's someone I want you to meet. This young man is my new associate, Dr. Humphreys."

I extended my hand and she met me with both of hers. Her hands were soft, but her grip was firm.

"It's a pleasure to meet you, Mrs. Zimmerman," I said.

"The pleasure is all mine, Dr. Humphreys." She smiled. "You're a lucky man to have such a wonderful teacher."

"Yes ma'am." I nodded. "Why don't I take Perky. I'll get him some fresh water. Nice meeting you, ma'am." I walked back to my office with the cage and placed it on my desk. I stepped back and examined the bird from a distance. He shivered, held his head down with his beak pressed against his breast, hidden under his wing. He ruffled his feathers to make himself look bigger, a classic defensive posture that most sick birds assume. The object is to *look bigger and maybe the bad guys will leave me alone*. He was in trouble.

After nearly fifteen minutes of flirting with Dr. T, Mrs. Zimmerman left. I was still evaluating a very sick bird when he stepped into our office.

"What do you think, young man?"

"I think he's looking for a place to die. How old is he?"

"Old enough to be on thin ice," he replied. "Let me have a look." He pulled his chair next to mine and began rolling up his sleeve. Was he really going to reach in and grab him? I thought—Bad idea. I kept quiet until he reached for the cage.

"Are you sure you want to do that, sir?" I asked, casually to disguise my concern. He stopped just before he opened the cage door and looked at me, puzzled. There was conflict in his eyes. Had I seen something that he had missed? That might be hard for him to take, I thought.

The truth was, I was familiar with this very situation. A few months earlier, I had an identical emergency call, a parakeet that teetered on his perch, his feathers ruffled, and his head buried under his wing. I needed to examine him and so, I reached into his cage and gently wrapped my hand around him. I removed him from his perch and his protective home. Like Perky, he too was looking for a place to die—I gave it to him. The stress of being handled was overwhelming and he died in my hand. Yes indeed, Dr. T. Reaching into that cage is a bad idea.

He withdrew his hand without saying a word. He stared at me with his usual hard look. Then the look softened. "What would you suggest?" he asked.

"I'm not sure anything is going to save him, sir," I said. "How about putting him on the counter in the bathroom and turning the shower on? Maybe if he breathes in a little steam, we can get him better hydrated—warm him up a bit?"

Then a rare sight—he smiled. "Okay. Sounds like a good plan. You get him set up. I'm going to mix up a little *yellow magic* to put in his water."

That was the second time I had heard reference to yellow magic. What in the world could that be?

I set the shower for full hot water. The staff bathroom was small and it didn't take long for the entire room to get hot and steamy. I left Perky to soak up some life-sustaining moisture until I exhausted the supply of hot water from the heater and the steam began to dissipate. I covered his cage with a thick blanket and returned him to my desk. Dr. T warmed a small dropper bottle in the palm of his hand while he waited for me. I watched as he counted ten drops of his magic yellow solution into the bird's water dish and covered the cage snuggly with the blanket.

I just had to know. "What is that stuff, Doc?"

"Someday, I just might tell you, young man," he said with a wicked smile. "I'm going home. See you after lunch."

I slipped into the treatment room where Tina, Laura, and Jack prepared to go on lunch break. Tina was our veterinary technician, a twenty-five-year-old single mother with short black hair, brown eyes and a perpetual smile that accentuated the dimples in her cheeks. She was shy and soft spoken, but confident and very good at her job. Laura and Jack were high school students and part-time employees. They were hard workers and great assistants to Tina.

Sixie sat on Tina's lap. He was the hospital cat, an overweight, grey tabby named for the six toes he had on both front feet. Sixie slept in the barn at night, but was allowed to wander the hallways during the day.

I waited until I heard the back door slam shut which indicated that Dr. T was gone and out of reach of our conversation.

"Okay, you guys," I said, rubbing my hands together. "What the heck is this yellow magic stuff?" They all looked at each other and then at me.

"Nobody knows, Dr. Humphreys. He won't let anyone see him mix it," Tina said.

"He locks the door to the lab when he's making a batch so nobody can see what he pulls off the shelf," Laura said. "Why do you think Polly calls him Dr. Jekyll?"

"He puts it on everything. I think I saw him pouring it into his coffee the other morning," Jack said.

6 – Yellow Magic

"Don't think it's made him any younger or wiser, do you?" I chuckled. "I'll see you guys after lunch."

The afternoon was busy. I ran from one exam room to the next and struggled to keep our little yellow friend out of my mind. I wanted to check on him, but I knew it was best not to disturb him any more than necessary. Before I knew it, the day was gone. I walked into our office and caught Dr. T peeking into Perky's cage through separated edges of the blanket.

"How's he doing?" I asked.

"I don't know. It's a bit early to say, but he sure doesn't look good."

"You got any other ideas?" I asked.

There was no response. He closed the edges of the blanket and meticulously tucked Perky in for the night. Finally, and without looking at me, he said, "You don't believe in my yellow magic, do you?"

"I didn't say that. I don't have a clue what it is."

"Trust me," he said and winked. "Those hotshot professors that supposedly taught you everything you'll ever need to know could learn a lesson or two from this old man."

"I don't doubt that a bit, sir," I said, although I wasn't sure I really agreed with him.

"It's been a long day. He'll be okay tonight." He sighed. "Let's go home."

I didn't sleep well that night. I thought of Mrs. Zimmerman and wondered how she would handle the loss of her buddy if Perky died. I arrived at the hospital the next morning and went straight to my office. On my desk set an empty cage and the blanket that once covered it, now neatly folded by its side. A single yellow feather lay on the floor in front of the cage.

I felt sick, but I wasn't surprised. I knew to expect this outcome. I turned to see four people looking through the open door to my office. Polly and Tina cried while Laura and Jack stood emotionless.

"Oh well, we knew his chances weren't very good. We gave it our best shot," I said. For a minute, there was silence.

"You haven't heard the complete story, Dr. Humphreys," Polly said.

"What do you mean?"

"I'm sorry, Dr. Humphreys," Tina sobbed. "I forgot to put Sixie out last night. Somehow, the hallway door was left open." Tina always made sure that Sixie was put outside for the night.

At first, I didn't understand what she was trying to say. Then I saw Tina's lips trembling and I felt a chill. "Wait a minute. Am I hearing this right? The damn cat ate the canary!" I asked, hoping I had misunderstood. Four heads nodded affirmatively. "Oh, shit!"

"He didn't eat him. Just chewed him up. I can't believe he did it, Dr. Humphreys. Sixie wouldn't hurt a fly," Tina said, still crying.

"Do you suppose Perky was already dead?" Polly asked. Just then, the phone rang. She ran to answer it.

"I think he was. I can't believe Sixie would have killed him," Tina said.

"Well, if he was still alive, seeing a twenty-pound kitty smiling outside his cage probably scared him to death," Laura said.

"Dead or alive, Sixie had him a little fun. Popped that bird's little head right off," Jack said with a silly grin.

"Gee, thanks for the details, Jack," I said with an emphatic glare that I trusted would accentuate my displeasure. I wrapped my arm around Tina. "Accidents happen, Tina. I'm with you. I think he was already dead."

Laura and Jack both whispered supportive words to Tina. She dried her tears. The back door opened and we heard approaching steps in the hallway. It was Dr. T.

"What in the hell is everybody doing standing around?" he hollered. Then he apparently noticed that something was wrong and his expression changed from anger to one of concern. "What's going on?"

"We have a problem, sir," I answered. I informed him of the unfortunate incident.

He stood motionless and stared at Tina for a long time. He didn't have to say anything. Tina saw the anger, the hatred in his eyes.

"Okay, people, let's get to work," he commanded. They all crept down the hallway to their respective hideaways.

"What do we do now?" I asked, hoping for some brilliant solution to correct a horrible accident.

He didn't respond for a long time. I could tell he struggled, trying to make sense of it all and was perhaps busy formulating a plan for our next move.

"I guess I'll have to tell her he died, won't I," he said with a deep sigh.

"You gonna give her any details?" I asked.

"What purpose would that serve?"

"None. For all we know, Perky was dead before Sixie got to him," I said.

Dr. T shook his head. From the look on his face, I felt certain he didn't believe that statement for a minute and it probably hurt him deeply that he would never know for sure. Had his yellow magic worked or not? Polly suddenly appeared at the door.

"That was Mrs. Zimmerman on the phone. The birthday party was wonderful, but she's anxious to get home. They're cutting their visit short. Should be here mid-afternoon to pick up Perky."

"Did you say anything to her?" Dr. T asked.

"Not in my job description."

"What if she asks to see the body?" I asked, having already experienced that nightmare.

"Well, I can't very well glue his little head back on, can I," Dr. T said. "I'll have to tell her I buried him. She'll be okay with that." He sighed. "There's something I gotta do. See you after lunch."

After lunch, I found Polly in a scurry, attempting to organize several things at once before running her errands.

"Dr. Humphreys, Mrs. Bailey just dropped off two cats to be spayed. I told her you'd get to them this afternoon. Dr. T has a horse waiting out back for a lameness exam. I have to take the deposit to the bank, but Lisa is going to cover for me until I get back." Lisa was

6 – Yellow Magic

Polly's teenage daughter, a senior in high school. She didn't have afternoon classes which freed her to fill in for her mother when Polly had errands to run.

"Your next appointment isn't for two hours," Polly said. "Should give you enough time to get caught up," she yelled as she ran out the door.

I walked into our office and found Dr. T busy at his desk. Next to him, in Perky's cage, a beautiful, tiny, yellow bird fluttered its wings and preened its feathers.

"What the hell is this," I exclaimed and pointed to the canary. Dr. T put his pen down and looked at me.

"A little gift. Maybe it'll help soften the blow of losing her little buddy." He shook his head, slowly. "She doesn't have anybody else," he said.

I was shocked. I saw a side of the man that, until now, I hadn't believed existed.

We had work to do. I heard Dr. T exit the back door on his way to examine the lame horse as I scrubbed my hands. Tina had the first cat anesthetized and on the table, ready for surgery. It took me an hour to spay both cats. As I peeled off my gloves, I heard a familiar yell in the distance. Dr. T must have finished with his exam of the lame horse, I thought. I ripped off my cap and mask and rushed down the hall, still in my surgery gown. Lisa had apparently heard the yell as well and she too, dashed down the hallway. Polly was still away running her errands. Lisa and I reached the doorway to Dr. T's office at the same time as the second yell echoed through the entire building.

"Where is the bird!" Dr. T searched his office in a panic.

"You mean Perky?" Lisa asked.

"Where are the cage and the bird?" he repeated with growing impatience.

"I sent him home," Lisa said.

"You did what?"

"I sent him home. Wasn't I supposed to?"

"When?" he asked, his hands on his hips.

"About a half hour ago. Mrs. Zimmerman came in with her neighbor. They were anxious to get home, so I helped her load him into the car. Don't worry, I sent the bag with all his stuff." Lisa said, her lips now trembling.

Just then, Polly entered the building and heard just enough to figure out what was going on. She had forgotten to tell Lisa that the bird was not to go home until Dr. T talked to Mrs. Zimmerman. Polly walked up behind her daughter and placed her hands on Lisa's shoulders.

"Thank you, sweetheart. Maybe you had better get home. I'll see you a little later." Lisa smiled sheepishly and hurried out the door.

Polly slipped around the corner to answer the phone. Dr. T and I sat down to confront our new problem. "This just gets better and better. What do we do now?" I asked.

Dr. T ran his fingers through his hair several times and buried his face in the palms of his hands. "Let me think about it for a bit," he said.

Polly finished her conversation and hung up the phone.

6 – Yellow Magic

"Polly," Dr. T yelled.

Within seconds, she was at his office door. She had a strange look on her face, not one of panic or concern, but rather a mysterious look, perhaps one of excitement and anticipation.

"Yes, sir?"

"Call Mrs. Zimmerman," he ordered. "Tell her I'm on my way to see her. Should be there in about twenty minutes." He paused. "On second thought, let me talk to her. I better be the one to tell her I'm coming."

"Yes, sir. I'll call her back," Polly said, with emphasis on *back*. She didn't move, hoping he would catch the ever so subtle hint. He did.

"What do you mean, call her back?"

"That was her I was just talking to," Polly said with a warm smile.

Dr. T's face suddenly froze with his eyes and mouth wide open. I had never seen him like this before. "What did she say?" he asked.

"Oh . . . the regular stuff. What a marvelous human being Dr. T is. Miracle worker. Knight in shining armor. You know," she said.

"Aaand?" he asked.

"Well, she did confess that Perky has been sick a lot longer than what she first told you. She didn't expect to see him alive again. He sang to her, all the way home."

"And?" he repeated, now with growing anticipation.

"I think that was all," Polly said. "Oh yeah. One more thing. She doesn't care what it costs. She wants two bottles of yellow magic, one for Perky and one for her. Shall I get her on the phone for you, sir?"

With interlaced fingers, he cradled the back of his head, leaned back in his chair, placed both feet on his desk, and looked up at the ceiling. That elusive smile stretched across his face.

"Let me think about it for a bit."

Chapter 7
LUCKY???

In the early spring of 1983, my employers, Dr. T and Dr. Mike dissolved their partnership. Dr. T retired. I bought his interest in the practice and fulfilled my dream to become a full partner in what would soon become one of the busiest veterinary practices in New Mexico. Mike and I built a new modernized hospital on a busy corner of town. As summer approached, the two of us headed into our busiest time of the year and faced the workload of three people. We were not prepared for the unexpected.

Tina agreed to continue working mornings. The rest of our new crew were young and inexperienced. Chrissie was a recent high school graduate who we hoped to groom to eventually take Tina's position. She assisted with daily treatments and surgeries, fed and watered both small and large animals, and cleaned cages. We hired her younger sister, Dee, to work that summer. Laura was our new receptionist. She had a long way to go to match Polly's experience and people skills, but she was a fast learner.

Tim was a twenty-five-year-old perpetual college student who had tried unsuccessfully for years to get into veterinary school. He had worked for us during summer months for the past several years. Tim was skinny as a toothpick, with long straight hair that hung over his eyes. He had a truly abrasive persona and an ego that would put a diva to shame.

Mr. and Mrs. Bronson arrived late one afternoon with Mr. Bronson's prized black stallion, Lucky. They were a crowd favorite at the fair parade every year with Lucky's signature prance, his long mane and tail, and Mr. Bronson's black cowboy outfit accented by silver button studs and cuff links.

"Tim," Mike yelled. "Go out back and check on that horse that just came in. Jim or I will join you as soon as we get caught up."

My last client of the afternoon had 101 questions about her dog, Buffy. With that task completed, I quickly changed into coveralls and headed to the large animal treatment room. The Bronsons, Chrissie, Dee, and Tim, together, managed to get Lucky into the stanchion—an open metal frame enclosure long enough to cage a single standing horse, yet narrow enough to provide proper restraint for examination or treatment.

Everyone watched Tim as he lifted the horse's upper lip and confidently spat out all kinds of information as he diagnosed his patient's illness. His job had never been more than to assist the rest of our crew and gain some experience that would hopefully aid him in his quest to get into veterinary school. As usual, he was way out of line. When I walked into the room, he stepped back, wiped Lucky's saliva from his face onto his shirt, and puffed up his chest.

"He's got *choke*, Doc," he declared. "Choke" refers to a horse that has an esophageal obstruction. It occurs when dry food travels down the esophagus toward the stomach and gets stuck mid-way, a painful ordeal for the horse.

Tim continued his show and as if under his spell, his audience crowded closer when he lifted the horse's head, grabbed his tongue, pulled it off to one side, and barked, "Chrissie, shine that flashlight into his mouth!" Five heads leaned toward each other, each anxious to be the first to look into Lucky's mouth. The horse coughed several times and sent a shower of droplets into the air and into the eyes and mouths of the clueless five.

I approached Lucky for a quick visual exam. A sense of uneasiness came over me. This horse wasn't sweating or acting as though he was in pain and contrary to Lucky's normal high-spirited demeanor, he appeared disoriented, unconcerned, or perhaps unaware of the chaotic activity that surrounded him. This wasn't normal.

Tim prepared a bucket of water, a stomach tube and pump, everything I needed to clear Lucky's esophageal obstruction.

"I got everything you need, Doc. I'll hold on to his halter while you pass the tube," he blurted with self-assuredness.

I stood directly in front of Lucky and looked into his eyes. I knew this horse well. He was a celebrity, and a prima donna. He craved the attention of an audience. He held a classic pose when he knew people were watching—his head high with perked ears, but not today. His eyes were blank, lost in a dream. He was undoubtedly sick and it quickly became apparent to me that this was no esophageal obstruction. Lucky's sickness was in his brain.

A sudden fright came over me, the memory, the admonishment, the written promise. The promise I made to a wonderful professor, Dr. Scrutchfield—*I will never examine a sick horse without first taking a minute to consider the possibility of rabies!* Now, I stood in a room with a horse showing what I believed to be neurological disease and five innocent people all covered in horse spit and completely oblivious to the fact that they might very well have just been exposed to one of the most horrible and deadly diseases on earth.

Rabies is a viral disease. All Rhabdoviruses are deadly. Under an electron microscope, they look very appropriately like bullets. Most exposures are the result of a bite wound, but salivary contact on an open wound, in the mouth, or in the eyes is sufficient exposure to cause disease. Once it's within the body, the virus travels by way of nerves to the spinal cord and eventually to the brain. Victims of the disease die a horrible death. The mortality rate is a hundred percent. That means, if you contract rabies, you're going to die.

"I'd like everybody to step away from the horse," I said, trying my best to remain calm.

"What do you mean?" Tim hissed in a defiant tone. He didn't like or respect me.

"I don't think this horse has choke, Tim. There's something else going on. You haven't given him any tranquilizer, have you?"

7 –Lucky???

"Tranquilizer? Of course not!" He sneered. "What do you mean something else?" I stared directly at him until I was certain I had made eye contact with him.

"I was thinking he just might have rabies." I said calmly. The room became quiet. Chrissie and Dee frantically wiped the saliva from their faces with the sleeves of their shirts. The Bronsons were speechless. Tim lacked the ability to control his tongue.

"Heh, you're kidding," he said with his signature smirk that I had grown to dislike.

"Oh, how I wish I was."

"What part of Dr. Humphreys' instructions don't you understand?" Mike had quietly entered the room and heard just enough to assess the situation.

"Move," he ordered.

Like a covey of quail, the suddenly not so fearless five lined up one behind the other and scurried toward Mike.

"Dr. Humphreys and I will handle it from here. I want everybody to go up front and wash your hands and face, now!" He turned to Mr. Bronson.

"How long's he been like this, Ted?" Mike asked.

"He was fine last night, Doc. He has a big pasture he plays in. When he wasn't waiting at the fence for his breakfast, I knew something was wrong. He just stood there in the middle of the field. I finally decided this afternoon to bring him in."

"Well, you and Mrs. Bronson might as well head home," Mike said. "We're going to check Lucky over carefully and I'll call you when we have some answers. It'll probably be tomorrow. I know he's your baby, Ted. We'll do everything we can for him."

There was a genuine look of fear on Mr. Bronson's face. He nodded without a word.

"Tim, show the Bronsons where the bathroom is," Mike said.

"Yes sir," Tim answered. The tone of his voice was more subdued. Mike looked at me and shook his head.

"I think he's neurological," I said.

"I'm sure you're right. Let's be careful," Mike replied.

We put on safety glasses, surgical masks, and long plastic gloves. We both understood the risk we were about to take. The safety measures were little more than a formality. If Lucky was rabid, we would consider ourselves exposed. I kept the horse's head as still as I could while Mike examined him. Lucky's pupils were non-responsive to light. He had trouble keeping his tongue in his mouth as if it were partially paralyzed and his muscles twitched wildly for no apparent reason.

"What do you think?" I asked.

"It's definitely neurological," Mike said. I saw the growing concern on his face.

"You don't suppose he's actually rabid, do you?" I asked.

"Probably not. Odds are he's got either St. Louis Encephalitis or Western Equine Encephalitis." His voice was calm, but not reassuring. "It's too late to get any blood to the lab tonight. The courier's come and gone."

"What do we do?" I asked.

7 –Lucky???

"Well, let's give him five liters of IV fluids and put him up for the night. If he's still alive tomorrow, we may have dodged a bullet."

"And if he's not?" I prayed for a reassuring answer.

"We'll have to cut his brain out and send it to the diagnostic lab," he said with a deep sigh.

As I drove home, I wondered whether to tell Katy or not. That question was quickly answered when Katy looked at my face.

"Uh oh. What happened?"

I tried to make light of the situation as I filled her in on the events of the day.

"Do you think he's rabid?" she asked.

"Naw. I agree with Mike. He either has W.E.E. or St. Louis E. I'm not too worried about it," I lied so as not to alarm her. "Worst-case scenario is that he dies. Lots of things could cause him to die, but we'll have no choice but to have his brain analyzed. If he's positive for rabies, we all have to get vaccinated."

"You mean those thirty shots in the belly?" Katy said with a grimaced face. So much for my efforts not to alarm her.

"No. It's different now. There's a newer vaccine, human diploid. Everyone gets a shot of immunoglobulin to give immediate protection. That one is a bit tough. The volume given is based on weight." I thought of the Bronsons, each weighing well over 200 pounds. Each would get a huge dose of expensive serum. The cost would be ours, but the pain, theirs. "Then we each get seven injections in the arm or the butt, three or four days apart," I continued. "The worst part will be the cost. Probably be a couple thousand dollars apiece. Insurance should cover most of it. It won't come to that. He'll be fine tomorrow," I said confidently with a smile.

I didn't sleep that night. I suspected that no one else had either.

When I arrived at work the next morning, I saw Mike standing beside a dead horse. I joined him and shared the silence and the wonder—what could we have done differently. Mike sighed.

"Poor Lucky wasn't so lucky after all," he said. "I'm pretty sure this wasn't rabies. Unfortunately, what I think, doesn't matter anymore."

Our focus had changed. Our priority was no longer to obtain a definitive diagnosis of what had killed Lucky, but rather to protect seven human beings who had possibly been exposed to rabies. The only way to be certain was to let the lab experts examine his brain.

"I'll take his head off as soon as we get caught up," Mike said. "Probably need some help cutting his brain out. There's a bone saw in the back room. Guess I better call Mr. Bronson. Sure not looking forward to this."

Mike called Mr. Bronson with the bad news. It was almost noon when we finally broke loose from the exam rooms.

"Let's get some lunch," Mike said. "We'll cut his brain out as soon as we get back." I was hungry and wasn't about to argue.

After lunch, we went to work on Lucky. With a sharp necropsy knife, Mike severed the head with ease. Next came the hard part, removing the hide and carefully sawing a window out of the top of Lucky's skull through which we would remove his brain.

7 –Lucky???

Arrangements were made to transport the rest of Lucky's body away for burial.

We prepared to start the unpleasant task of removing Lucky's brain when our receptionist, Laura, appeared at the back door. "Dr. Mike, Ben Thompson just called. He has a horse with colic. He needs you out there right away."

"Don't worry. I can do this," I said.

"No, you can't," Laura said. "Luiz Dairy called right after Mr. Thompson. They have a cow trying to calve. Sounds like you may be doing a C-section." There was little time to think about anything.

"Call Public Health in Albuquerque. Tell them we're sending them a brain. Rabies suspect! On the bus. Tonight," Mike yelled. He looked at me.

"Get back here as soon as you can." We moved Lucky's head into the shade of a tree, climbed into our vehicles, and sped out the gate in opposite directions.

I arrived at the dairy just as the foreman and one of his workmen were delivering the calf. Maybe our luck is finally changing, I thought. I examined the cow, infused her uterus with a disinfectant solution, loaded up my equipment, and raced back to the office. Mike had arrived ahead of me. I walked into our office as he hung up the phone.

"Are you ready?" he asked.

"Let's get it done," I said. To our relief, the horse's body had been picked up. We walked toward the big tree where we had placed the head earlier and then, what we thought was already a lousy day, just got worse.

"Where the hell is the head?" Mike yelled.

Goose bumps raced up my arms. The head was gone!

"I don't know," I said, still confident there must be an explanation. "Surely, they wouldn't have taken the head, would they?" I didn't expect an answer and became increasingly alarmed. Suddenly, Tim appeared from around the corner.

"Tim," Mike yelled. Tim yawned. He looked like his noon nap had just been rudely interrupted.

"What," he yelled back.

Mike looked left, then right, desperate for an answer.

"Where's the damn head," he repeated.

"What?" Tim started a full speed run toward us, then stopped, and stared. "I swear, Dr. Mike, I was right here when they picked up the horse." His voice trembled with fear. "The head was right there when they left." He pointed to a bloody spot at the base of the tree. "Really—right there!"

There had to be an answer, I thought. I frantically scanned the entire yard and searched for clues. Then I saw the empty space in the corner of the yard—the green pickup was gone. "Shit!" I ran as fast as I could toward the office building. Laura, Chrissie, and Dee hovered around the receptionist's desk and chatted as if they had not a care in the world. I was out of breath.

"Does anyone know where Jon Boy is?" I cried out.

"Jon Boy?" Laura said. "He got here about an hour ago. I think he's out back."

7 – Lucky???

His name was Jonathan Myers, but he was Jon Boy to all of us. He was a high school student who had worked for us for the past three years. This tall thin cowboy came in three afternoons a week after school and on an occasional weekend if the girls had a personal activity going on. He fed and watered the animals, cleaned, painted, and did anything necessary to keep the place looking nice. We loved this kid. He was a genuine pleasure to have around. More importantly, Jon Boy knew his job well. He didn't wait to be told what to do. If he saw something that didn't look right, he fixed it.

"Pretty sure he was going to bag up the trash and take it to the dump," Dee said.

I was halfway down the hallway before she finished her sentence. I ran out the door and screamed, "Mike!"

Mike had figured out the puzzle as well. He was already in his pickup. His back tires spit gravel into the air as they dug for traction. He was out the gate in a cloud of dust in hot pursuit of Jon Boy. He didn't make it very far before he passed the young man, returning from the landfill with an empty truck.

Jon Boy came through the gate with Mike on his back bumper. They stepped out of their trucks. With blood-stained hands, shirt, and pants, Jon Boy looked at three anxious faces. "What?" he asked.

Mike took a deep breath and asked in a calm voice, "Jon Boy, did you see the horse's head that was under the tree?"

"Of course I did," Jon Boy answered confidently. "I wasn't gonna just leave it there collecting flies all afternoon. Don't worry, Dr. Mike.

I double-bagged it so the guy at the dump wouldn't bitch," he said with a smile.

Double bagging a bleeding, saliva-ridden horse's head made Jon Boy the newest member of the exposed club—*and then there were eight.*

"I stuck around to make sure the bull-dozer buried it good and deep before I left," Jon Boy said proudly. Mike, Tim, and I stood with bowed heads as if in silent prayer for a few seconds.

"I'll call the lab," I said and started walking across the yard. When I reached the back door to the main building, I looked over my shoulder. Jon Boy stood alone, his hands covering his face, and sobbed.

Mike put his arms around the young man and held him tightly. He had done what he thought was right and what was expected of him. He was used to picking up the body parts after we delivered a dead calf or finished a post-mortem exam on a dead sheep or pig. Why should a horse's head be any different? It was his job to keep the place clean and he did it well. He had made a huge mistake, he knew it, and there was nothing he could do to change that.

Without any verbal reprimand from Mike or me, he now bore the burden of knowing how costly his mistake was and yet, there was never any doubt that the responsibility for this crazy accident rested solely with Mike and me.

Mike drove to the landfill and pleaded with the dozer operator to dig up the head. "Impossible," he was told.

7 –Lucky???

In the meantime, it was my duty to call the public health department who expected a brain on the late bus.

"You did what?" the state epidemiologist asked in a disbelieving tone.

"You heard me right, Doc," I said. "Our brain is buried under several tons of dirt."

There was a silence that followed and I wondered, is he struggling to control his laughter or is he writing down notes that he will later present to the board of veterinary examiners in hopes that they will have the good sense to revoke my license? He finally broke the silence.

"Do you really think he was rabid?" he asked.

"I guess what I think, is irrelevant, isn't it?" I hoped the tone of my voice would properly express my irritation at his question.

"Get me accurate body weights on everybody exposed," he said without hesitation. "I need to talk to your private physician. I'll see if he or she is willing to administer the vaccinations. We'll have the state police carry the vaccine down to you tomorrow morning. You should have it by noon. Any questions?"

"No, sir." I felt like a kid who had just been caught painting graffiti on the neighbor's front door.

The more difficult tasks were yet to come. I gave the Bronsons a second dose of bad news. Then I called two sets of parents and tried to explain why, even though we really didn't know for sure why this horse had died, their kids had no choice but to endure the misery of rabies shots.

Over the next few weeks, the eight of us underwent a grueling schedule of post-exposure treatment for rabies. Everyone survived. The total cost of the treatment was many thousands of dollars. Insurance paid for most of it. Mike and I paid the rest.

To our surprise, the Bronsons continued to be loyal clients for years. Chrissie and Dee decided that anything was better than working at a veterinary hospital. Chrissie enrolled in college and Dee decided to take up cheerleading. Jon Boy continued to work for us until the day he graduated. We always remembered him as one of the best.

As for Tim—that summer was the last we ever saw of him. Not a phone call, nor a letter. He simply vanished. Sometime later, we heard a rumor that he had decided to go to law school, a wise choice, indeed.

We all learned a valuable lesson that fateful day. Even so, it was years before I could call the diagnostic lab inquiring about results on a sample we had submitted without having to listen to their clichéd response—"Oh, yeah. You guys are the ones who lost the horse's head, right?"

Chapter 8

BANJO

Monday mornings were always busy. The hospital was usually full of emergency cases that had been taken in over the weekend. Some still required intensive care. Thankfully, we now had Diane on staff. She was our new assistant who took care of our small animal patients.

We had just finished with the morning treatments when our receptionist, Laura, burst into the treatment room and looked up at the ceiling as if asking heaven for forgiveness.

"There's a lady on the phone with a sick dog. He's too sick to bring in, so she needs somebody to go out to her place. Oh yeah, and he bites," Laura added.

My partner, Mike, looked up from a patient record he was finishing. "Hey, you know I'd go, but Mrs. Johnson is bringing Beau in to see me," he said as he grinned from ear to ear. He looked at the clock. "She's due any minute."

"Yeah, I know," I said. I turned to Laura. "Tell her I'm on my way."

"I'll get directions for you," she said as she ran out the door.

I followed her to the reception desk. "Who is this lady?" I asked Laura as I wrote down directions.

"I have no idea. We've never seen her or any of her animals before. She sounds very nice. Diane has two dentals this morning, so you'll have to take Santiago."

Santiago was our large animal assistant. He was used to dealing with cows and horses, but I knew he could handle a mean dog or anything else I asked of him.

Santiago was born in Mexico and came to the United States as a ten-year-old boy. He was hard-working, smart, skilled, honest, and had one serious problem—he was undocumented. By the time he came to us, he was married to a U.S. resident and had two sons, both American citizens—facts that were of no consequence to the Immigration and Naturalization Service. To make things worse, Santiago had been deported on three separate occasions, a serious blemish on his immigration record. Nevertheless, with the support of a sympathetic congressman, we engaged in a long-term battle with the INS.

"Where are we going, *patrón*?" Santiago asked. Although I was his boss, I considered Santiago a friend and asked him repeatedly to call me by my first name. Occasionally he did, but generally, he adhered to the Mexican tradition of addressing the boss in the respectful way—*patrón*.

"We've got a sick dog. Apparently, he's not very nice so you better bring a good leash and a muzzle."

My company truck was basically a veterinary ambulance designed for large animal emergencies. It had a fiberglass shell that fit snugly in the bed of the truck and was equipped with a temperature controlling system, hot and cold running water, a refrigerator, and drawers that held just about any drug or piece of equipment necessary to treat a horse, cow, pig, or sheep. Because we weren't often called to handle a small animal emergency outside of the office, this call required a bit more planning. I threw everything I could think of into a black bag.

Santiago was a short man who walked tall. He took pride in his appearance and always looked dapper with his neatly pressed tucked-in shirt, creased blue jeans, and spit-shined boots that looked like mirrors on his feet. He was always clean-shaven, sporting only a trimmed mustache, the signature of a proud Mexican gentleman.

Laura's directions were far from perfect, as was often the case. "Turn right at the railroad tracks" was supposed to be a left turn. We wandered around for the better part of thirty minutes. We weren't lost, we just weren't sure of where we were. Cell phones and GPS were dreams of the future at the time. We finally came upon a place that we hoped was where we were supposed to be.

In front of us was a large open field with no grass, no trees, and no neighbors. In the distance was a dilapidated trailer that looked like it could easily be brought to the ground by the next heavy windstorm. For as far as I could see, the field was littered with parts—car parts, tractor parts, washer and dryer parts, toilet parts, parts that looked like they belonged in a museum, and parts that didn't seem to belong to anything.

Behind the trailer was a strange looking building with wooden walls and a tin roof. It was about ten feet wide, ten feet high, and half the length of a football field running north and south. There were no windows, some skylights, air vents, and double barn doors at the north end. Attached to the south end was a six-foot high chain link fence that surrounded a one-acre field of planted corn. It was thick with seven-foot-high stalks that had been allowed to dry. In the center of the near side of the fence was a wide gate, chained and locked.

Santiago and I stepped out of the truck. An elderly woman appeared at the door of the trailer. She wore a plaid shirt and blue jeans pulled up to her ribs and cinched tightly with a belt that was a foot too long. She grimaced as she struggled to walk down the steps to greet us.

"Are you Dr. Humpy?" A broad smile revealed two upper teeth that hung on precariously to unhealthy looking gums.

"Uh, yes ma'am, I'm Dr. Humphreys."

"My baby's awful sick, Doc," she said. "He hasn't answered the breakfast or dinner bell for three days. It's just not like him. I'm plum worried sick about him."

I expected to see an old flea-ridden mangy dog crawl out from under the trailer. I scanned the area and found no clues. "So, where is he, ma'am? I'm sorry, what is your name again?" I asked.

"I'm Florence," she said with a shallow bow. "Florence Gibbs, but you can call me Flo. His name is Banjo and he's out there." She pointed to the fenced cornfield.

There was a pause in the conversation as I looked and wondered what I had gotten myself into. "Okay," I said. I pointed to the locked gate. "Is that how we get in, Mrs. Gibbs?"

"Nope. I lost the key. We'll have to go through the coop, Doc, and please, call me Flo."

"Yes ma'am. I mean, Flo. So, tell me a bit about Banjo, Flo. Is he mean?"

"Well, it's like I told your girl at the office, Doc. He likes to bite, but his bite ain't half as bad as his kick."

"His kick?" I asked. What kind of dog kicks, I wondered, and how am I supposed to find a biting, kicking dog in that mass of corn stalks?

"Yes sir," she replied. "He's a big rascal and it don't matter where you're standing. If you're close enough to put a hand on him and he gets to feelin' a bit frisky, he can put his back foot in your hip pocket before you can count to . . . well, real fast."

"Mrs. Gibbs, I mean Flo, what kind of dog is Banjo?" I was now totally confused and disturbed.

"Dog?" She looked at me as if I had asked if the sun truly rose in the east. "Banjo ain't no dog. He's my mule!"

"What!" I was shocked for a moment. Then it hit me. *Laura!* Why can't you get anything straight? I turned toward Santiago who was bent over, laughing.

"Put that stupid leash away," I snarled. "Get your rope."

Of all his skills, Santiago had one that stood out well above the rest—he was a great roper. He could rope the hind legs of a flying gnat. I stared at the jungle of dried corn we were about to enter. Gnats have nothing to worry about today, I thought. I forced a smile and turned to look at Flo. "This could be a challenge." A challenge, I thought. Really? Maybe more like a suicide mission.

"Don't think he'll give you any trouble, Doc," Flo said. "He must be awful sick. I just hope he ain't dead." Dead? That just might be a blessing, I thought.

"Okay, let's give it a go," I said as I fought to hang on to my smile.

Santiago prepared his rope. He formed a loop and started a controlled swing over his head, slow at first, then faster and faster until he reached a rhythm. It was a beautiful thing to watch Santiago and his rope. In short time, he and the rope were synchronized. Without warning, he suddenly cast the swinging loop into the air. With the precision of a guided missile, it floated, floated, and then landed directly on its target. He drew the rope tightly and smiled, having roped one of Flo's decorative washing machines.

"I'm ready," he said, bubbling with confidence.

We headed toward the north end of the building as Santiago retrieved his rope.

"What is this building, Flo, and why do you call it the coop?" I asked.

"It's my coop, Doc," she said as she reached for the doors, "and these are my girls." The doors flew open and there it was—the largest, noisiest, and most compact collection of birds I had ever seen or heard. A narrow alley was flanked by four rows of cages on either side, stacked one upon the other, the entire length of the coop. Each cage held a single hen, some white, some black, some brown. Each bird poked her head out of a narrow slot in the cage, designed perhaps to give her the feeling that escape was, possible.

The air was thick with the smell of chicken manure. Down feathers floated everywhere like snowflakes. The noise was deafening and yet, it had a special quality, like a choir of content chickens. I noticed several free flying fowl.

"How come these chickens aren't caged, Flo?" I asked.

She turned toward me with a look of disbelief. "Are you kiddin' me, Doc? Those are my roosters!"

"Oh yeah," I said as I attempted to disguise my ignorance.

"Hey, look who's here!" exclaimed Flo. Directly in front of us, towering and still as a statue, was a beautiful rooster. His comb was tall and cherry red. Even the dim light could not hide his large full breast and his brilliantly colored feathers which shone like a rainbow.

"This is Ringo, Doc. He's my best boy. Ain't he a beauty?" Flo asked proudly.

I wasn't much of an expert on or even the slightest bit interested in chickens. I might never have noticed Ringo, but there was something special about this rooster. He strutted with a certain panache. His great looks and cocky attitude said, *Don't mess with me! I'm king of the coop*. I was impressed.

"Been offered a lot of money for him," Flo said. "No way I could ever let him go. He's pretty special."

"He is indeed," I said.

We continued down the hall and finally arrived at the south end of the coop, the entrance to the world that belonged to Banjo. Flo threw open the double doors. All that could be seen was a solid wall of dried corn stalks.

"He's out there somewhere, Doc," she said.

"Maybe you had better wait here, Flo. If you would, shut the doors behind us," I said. I looked toward the solid mass of weeds in front of me. What were the odds of finding anything dead *or* alive out there? Not good. I glanced behind me and saw Santiago surveying the situation. He didn't have the answer either. Even if we did find him, what then? Santiago would have to find a way to get a rope around his neck, an easy task in wide-open spaces, but not so easy when surrounded by corn stalks that were two feet taller than he was.

My instincts told me to turn around and go home. *This is crazy.* Then I looked at Flo. Her face was full of emotion. On the surface, deep concern for Banjo, but also a smile and perhaps a ray of hope and trust in me. We were committed. There was nothing else to do but shuffle through the maze of maize in hopes of flushing out this big bad ass.

We moved ahead, step by step, and parted the stalks in front of us. We heard the stomping of hooves and cracking of the corn to our left, then to our right, and straight ahead, signaling that Banjo was very much aware of our presence and jockeying for position. We tracked the sounds of his movement. My heart beat faster. Sweat ran down my back. Santiago readied his rope. All was quiet and then I leaned forward, split the stalks directly in front of me, and came face to face with the large pink muzzle of the beast.

His eyes were black as night, his pupils dilated. He laid his ears back, flared his nostrils, snorted, and brayed, announcing that the games would begin. The gravity of our situation had not yet sunk in when he lunged forward. His broad chest caught me squarely on my left shoulder and tossed me to the ground like a billiard ball shot into a corner pocket. He ran past me. With only a second to give warning, I shouted, "Santiago!"

My partner saw the 1,000-pound projectile headed directly at him and jumped out of the way as the thunderous hooves stomped past him. The wide path of crushed corn stalks that Banjo left behind made him easier to follow. He can't go very far, I thought. He'll have to stop when he reaches the coop. Dear God, please get Flo out of the way!

"I'm on him!" Santiago yelled as he struggled to swing his rope in the air and raced after the beast. For a moment, I thought he might succeed. That twinkle of hope was quickly dashed. Flo had left a gap in the south doors, just wide enough for Banjo to see a way out. He hit the doors at full speed and never broke stride. The sound of splintering wood filled the air and I heard Flo yell, "You son of a bitch!"

Banjo entered the coop like a runaway freight train. His massive shoulders and butt crashed back and forth off the walls as he rumbled down the alley. Each time he hit a wall, cages were crushed while others fell to the ground. The necks of those hens, too slow to withdraw their heads into their protective cages, snapped like dried twigs. A few of the non-caged birds took flight in time to get up and over the top of the mule. Others were not so lucky.

Still stunned, I sat on the ground where the mule had planted me and listened to the squawking and screaming of chickens as Banjo galloped down the middle of the coop with Santiago in hot pursuit, trying to spin his rope through a sea of feathers.

When the mule finally reached the north end of the coop, he saw a gap in those doors and took them out as well. Like a ghost, he was gone. I picked myself off the ground and suddenly remembered—Flo! I stumbled toward the coop and found her, motionless. She sat with her back against the remnants of the south wall, mouth wide open, the last of her teeth still in place.

"Are you okay, Flo?" I asked.

She sighed. "I guess I shoulda' shot that stupid mule a long time ago."

I was relieved that she appeared to be unhurt. "Let me help you up," I said. We looked into the coop, shocked by the devastation. Slowly, we trekked down the path of carnage left by the beast. The air was thick with feathers. Chickens, some crushed, others headless, lay lifeless everywhere. Some of the loose birds were trampled into the dirt while others hung from the rafters. The floor, the walls and ceiling were all painted with blood. The cacophony of high-pitched squawks was now reduced to a chorus of pitiful moans as the survivors mourned the less fortunate.

I worried about Flo. What this poor woman had just witnessed was surely life changing. Just when it seemed that all was lost, a familiar figure appeared through the cloud of dust and debris. His majestic colors shone brightly, his feathers were untouched, and his ever-present royal strut persisted despite the apocalyptic picture that surrounded him.

"Ringo!" Flo yelled as she fell to her knees and embraced her best boy. The rooster was not quite as enthusiastic about this reunion and he let Flo know so with a firm peck to her head.

Santiago appeared at the north entrance to the coop. His shirt, soaked with sweat, was no longer tucked in. The lower half of his pants and his boots were covered in chicken blood and chicken shit. Feathers clung to his hair, his eyebrows, and his pristine mustache as if he had just lost a pillow fight. His rope lay limp on the ground and dragged behind him.

"Sorry, *patrón*," he said as he struggled to catch his breath. "He was too fast. That mule is crazy." Together, we helped Flo walk out of the coop.

"Flo, I don't know what to say," I said with both empathy and embarrassment.

"Aw, don't worry, Doc. At least I know he's all right. When he gets good and hungry, he'll be back."

I looked at her in disbelief. Her coop is in shambles, perhaps dozens of her "girls" were dead, and she was still worried about that idiot mule.

"Let us help you clean up this mess," I said.

"No, no, no," she said. "I'll call my grandsons. They'll take care of everything. Tell me what I owe you, Doc. I'll go get my checkbook."

There was no way I could add to the calamity that this sweet lady had just suffered and live with myself. "Oh, let's just call this one even, Flo. Are you sure we can't help you?" I asked as I looked desperately for some way to compensate this poor lady for her loss.

"You get on your way, Doc. Thanks for all your help," she replied.

Santiago and I walked to the truck, stepped inside, and shut the doors. I looked at him as if I had been awakened from a bad dream. "Can you believe what just happened?"

He broke into a broad smile and blew away a floating feather. *"Así es la vida, patrón. I love this job!"* With that, we drove away.

Chapter 9
TIME FOR A BABY?

Our Saturday mornings were typically lazy when I wasn't on call. Katy and I had just finished breakfast when the phone rang.

"Hey, what are you guys doing this evening?" It was my buddy, Jay. His great uncle had recently passed away. He and Dana were now married and had moved from their home in town, out to the ranch. In the short three years that I had known him, Jay blossomed from an inexperienced, unqualified urban cowboy to a hardened, well-seasoned rancher. He learned his trade the hard way—by trial and error. He worked tirelessly, employed good help, listened intensely to advice given, and took nothing for granted. On the weekends, he treated himself to a little time off.

"No plans that I know of, Jay. What's up?" I asked.

"You're not on call, are you?" I got the impression from his voice that if I were on call, the deal was off.

"No, thank goodness," I replied.

"Good. I'm gonna burn some ribs. Why don't you guys come over about six?"

"We'll bring a salad," I said. "See you at six."

Jay's ranch bordered the edge of town and was only six miles from our house. The first four were paved. The final two, a well-maintained private dirt road flanked by fenced pastures on either side, led to the headquarters.

The sun hung low on the horizon, partially cloaked by a thin wisp of pink stratus clouds as we drove south. To the right, as far as the eye could see, was a field of wheat grass speckled with Brangus cows, black as coal, as they grazed contently in the calm of their nature.

"Wow. Look at that," Katy said. "The sun setting over a carpet of green covered by fat, shiny cows. I love the desert."

"Me too," I said as I looked over her shoulder. "That's why we came back to New Mexico, right?"

I slowed down as pavement gave way to dirt. Katy sat silent and opened her senses to the colors, the aromas, and sounds of the evening.

"Jim, what's the matter with that cow?" she asked abruptly.

"What? What are you talking about?"

"That cow. Why is she all by herself?" She pointed out the window.

"Aw, don't worry about her. I'm sure she's fine," I replied.

"No. No, she's not. Stop the car."

I stopped and looked across the field.

"There," she said and pointed.

Just inside the fence line, separated from the rest of the herd, a single, fat heifer walked in tight circles, laid down, got up, walked in tight circles, and laid down again.

9 – Time for a Baby?

"This must be Jay's pregnant heifer pasture. She may be looking for place to calve," I said.

"Maybe we'd better wait here and see if she's going to need any help," Katy said as she gripped my knee.

"Don't be silly, sweetie," I chuckled. "Heifers have been calving on their own for lots of years. Besides, it could be hours before she goes into labor and they typically do better without somebody hovering over them. We gotta go. Jay and Dana are waiting for us." Reluctantly, Katy agreed.

The smell of ribs on the grill filled the air. "Hi, you guys," Dana yelled out the kitchen window. "Katy, I've got a margarita for you. Jay's out back, Jim. Beer is in the cooler."

"Thanks, Dana," I said with a smile.

"Tell Jay about the cow, okay," Katy whispered.

Music blared through outdoor speakers mounted on the wall of the back porch. Jay stood over a smoking grill with a beer in one hand and a long fork in the other as he sang along to Elton John's "Captain Fantastic."

"Do you know what you're doing?" I asked.

"Jim! How the hell are ya? Grab yourself a beer." He looked at his watch. "Ribs will be done in ten minutes."

"God, that smells good," I said. "Good music, too."

"Really? Been thinkin', maybe I need to start listening to country," Jay said. "You know, now that I'm a genuine cowboy and all?"

"Don't you dare," I said as I pointed my finger at him. "We rockers need to stick together. Besides, you may be a helluva rancher, but you're still a ways from being a cowboy. By the way, Katy spotted a heifer just north of the house when we came in. Looks like she may be calving soon. Katy's worried about her." I chuckled.

Katy appeared at the door of the back porch. Jay winked at me. "Don't worry about that heifer, Katy. She and another dozen or so are due any time. Tell you what. We'll take a drive after supper and peek in on her."

Katy took a deep breath, smiled, and walked back inside.

"I'll be done in five, Dana," Jay yelled as he flipped his signature ribs one last time. I reached into the cooler for a second round of beers.

We ate on the back porch. The weather was perfect. A gentle breeze kept the bugs at bay. Jay's ribs melted in our mouths. Dana's potato salad complimented wonderfully and Katy's mixed green salad was a delightful palate cleanser. The wine was the perfect accent to a relaxing evening.

"I am stuffed," Jay said with a deep sigh. "Has everybody had about as much fun as you can stand? Why don't we cram into my pickup and take a drive through the heifer pasture? I'm gonna put on some pants and boots, just in case."

"Jim, you want some clothes?" he asked.

I hadn't expected to walk through a hay field. I was dressed for a relaxing evening, shorts, a baby blue t-shirt, and sandals. "Naw, I'll be okay," I said.

It was dark when Jay pulled up to the gate of the pasture. I jumped out of the truck, opened the gate, and shut it as Jay drove through.

"Where is she, Katy?" Jay asked.

9 – Time for a Baby?

"She was over in that corner." Katy pointed straight ahead. The light of the bright moon illuminated the fence line, but the shapes of black cows blended easily into the night. Jay drove slowly until the headlights of the truck shined on reflective eyes. A heifer lay on her side, twenty feet from the fence and facing us.

The truck crept forward, slowly.

"That's Diamond," Dana exclaimed.

"Oh, shit," Jay said. He shook his head.

"Diamond?" I asked. "Her name is Diamond?" I looked across the seat at Dana. "How do you know she's Diamond?"

Then I turned to Jay. "What do you mean, *'oh, shit?'"*

"See that white spot on her neck below her chin? Looks like a diamond necklace," Jay said and sighed. "Dana named her. I've been trying to get rid of her. No self-respecting Brangus breeder has a cow with a white spot on her. It's embarrassing."

"She's beautiful. And, she's mine," Dana said.

"Oh, yeah? Well, you can have her," Jay said. "There's one more thing, Jim." He grinned. "She's not very nice."

Suddenly, I regretted having said anything to Jay about a heifer that might be in labor.

The truck was within twenty feet of Diamond when she rose onto her chest and shook her head nervously. She remained prone, but shifted her body ninety degrees. Just under the base of her tail, two tiny feet poked out of her birth canal.

"Uh oh," I said. Immediately, I felt uneasy. I sensed that Diamond might be in trouble.

"What?" Katy asked.

"She's calving," Jay said.

We sat in silence and watched for a minute.

"What do you think, Jim?" Jay asked.

"Well, we could just leave her alone and tomorrow morning, we'll probably find her nursing a healthy calf." I paused. "On the other hand, if that baby is too big or isn't positioned right, by tomorrow, it'll be dead, and Diamond will be one sick mama."

Jay took a deep breath. "Okay, let's pull that sucker," he said.

"You got what we need?" I asked.

"Yup. There's a rope, some OB chains, and handles in the back. You think we can sneak up behind her? If you can tie a rope off to the fence and toss me the free end, I'll try to throw a loop over her head."

"Sounds like a plan," I whispered.

"Maybe you girls should stay put for a bit," I suggested as we quietly climbed out of the pickup.

"Don't hurt her," Dana said.

I reached into the bed of the truck and found the rope. We gave Diamond a wide berth as Jay and I crept toward the fence. Although the field was clear of stickers and cactus, I regretted not to have accepted Jay's offer for long pants or a pair of shoes. The fence was constructed of three strands of barbwire supported every 25 feet by a mesquite post buried 30 inches into the ground. I selected the post closest to Diamond and tied the end of the rope with a clove hitch backed up by a double half-hitch. If Jay could get a noose around her neck, Diamond wasn't going anywhere.

9 – Time for a Baby?

The heifer looked over her shoulder at us, snorted, but didn't get up. Jay waited until she looked away. "Toss me the rope," he whispered.

As quietly as I could, I threw the free end of the rope to him. Jay caught it, formed a loop, and walked slowly toward the calving heifer. When he was as close as he felt he could get without disturbing her, he threw the loop into the air. It landed directly over the heifer's head. Jay drew the rope tightly on her neck.

"Got 'er, Jim," he said excitedly.

"Grab the OB chains, Jay." I now stood between Diamond and the fence. I used the rope to guide me and walked as fast as my sandals would allow toward the heifer. Then, much to my dismay, I felt the rope begin to tighten. Diamond stood up and moved away from the fence. The rope drew tighter. Then I heard a loud spine-tingling—*Crack! Crack! Crack!* What the hell was that, I wondered and suspected the worst.

"Jim! She's taking the fence with her. *Run,*" Jay yelled.

The mesquite post that the rope was tied to snapped at the ground, followed by the next one to the right and then the left. Diamond was on the move, dragging the fence directly toward me.

I heard the sound of splintered mesquite posts and rusty barbed wire as they ripped through the furrows of wheat grass headed in my direction—and closing fast. I started to run. My right foot stepped into a hole that pulled the sandal off my foot. I ran another ten feet and stepped on something slimy, perhaps a piece of placenta shed by Diamond. My foot slipped back out from under me and I flew forward in a swan dive. My hands reached out to break the fall. My chest hit the ground with a distinctive splat. The cow manure I landed on was moist, mushy, and smelly. I lay there, certain I would soon feel the wrath of barbed wire rake across my back. Suddenly, Diamond stopped, dropped to her chest, and rolled to her side. The weight of the fence had tired her and the adjacent posts had held.

"Are you okay," Jay yelled.

"Yeah," I said as I struggled to catch my breath. "Bring the OB chains, Jay." I used the rope to pull myself off the ground onto my knees and crawled toward Diamond. Her uterine contractions were much stronger now and they distracted her from imminent threat.

I reached her just as Jay arrived with the chains. Gently, I pulled on one of the exposed feet. Instinctively, the calf jerked the foot away from me.

"Calf's alive, Jay," I said. I reached both of my hands into the birth canal, confirmed that the exposed feet were indeed front feet, and found the calf's nose in position and ready to be delivered.

"We've got a head and two front feet. This baby is ready to meet the world." I looped a chain around each of the exposed feet and pulled them tightly. I reached deeper and felt the size of the calf's head.

"It's a big calf, Jay," I said. "May take both of us to get it out. You don't have a calf puller, do you?"

"No." Jay shook his head in disgust. "Wait a minute. I've got an idea." He ran to the truck, reached into the bed, and pulled out a logging chain.

9 – Time for a Baby?

"Dana," he yelled, "Drive the truck around directly behind Diamond!"

"What are you doing?" I asked. He handed me one end of his chain.

"Hook your OB chains onto this," Jay said. Dana moved the truck into position as instructed. Jay threaded his chain around the front bumper of the truck until there was no slack between it and the OB chains. I now understood the plan.

"Shove over, Dana," Jay said. He stepped into the pickup, started the engine, shifted into reverse, and leaned out the window. "You ready, Jim?"

I checked again to make sure the calf's feet and head were still in position and gave Jay a thumbs-up signal. "Take it slow, Jay."

He released the clutch, slowly. The chains held. The bumper held. Diamond's calf began a journey from the comfort of a warm, protective bubble, pulled through the tight squeeze of a narrow tunnel, out into the uncertainty of a brave new world. I watched as the head appeared. Then shoulders, chest, pelvis and finally, back legs fell out onto a cool bed of grass.

"That's good, Jay," I yelled and signaled with the wave of my hand.

I applied several chest compressions to clear the residual mucus from the calf's trachea, then wiped its nose and mouth. The calf coughed and shook its head. Jay jumped out of the pickup, loosened the rope, and removed the noose from around Diamond's neck.

Exhausted from the energy expended, but free of the pain of delivering an enormous calf, her muscles relaxed, and her breathing eased.

"Okay, you guys. Let's get things wrapped up and get the hell outta here while we're still welcome," Jay said. He reached into the bed of the pickup, grabbed two metal t-posts and a sledgehammer.

"Dana, will you give me a hand?" he asked.

"Katy, there's a towel behind the seat. Why don't you help Jim get the calf dried off?"

Diamond's calf began to breathe on its own. In the distance, I heard Jay and Dana as they hammered t-posts into the ground to reset the fence. Katy dried the calf's face while I removed the chains from its front legs. Diamond slowly rolled onto her chest.

"Watch her, sweetie," I said.

"He's a bull, Jay," I called out as I looked between the calf's back legs. "And a big rascal," I exclaimed, in awe of this calf that was close to twice the size of the average.

"Great! Just what I need. A big-ass bull with his mother's bad-ass attitude," Jay yelled back.

"Yay! I'm going to call him Prince," Dana yelled.

Prince rested on his chest and his mama gained more and more strength by the minute. It was time for us to leave. We gathered at the truck. Jay stopped and sniffed the air several times. "What stinks?" he asked.

"Uh, that would be me," I said.

9 – Time for a Baby?

The headlights shone on my new blue t-shirt, now tie-dyed, covered by a perfect bullseye of cow shit green. Jay lowered his gaze to my feet.

"Where are your sandals?" he asked.

"Haven't got a clue."

He laughed. "Don't worry. I'll find them tomorrow." He broke into a wide smile. "Why is it nothing we do together ever seems to come easy?"

"Aw, where's the fun in easy? I'll ride in the back," I said.

Back at the ranch house, Jay gave me a change of clothes.

"Thank you so much, guys," Katy said. "The evening was wonderful. Jay, if you'll let me borrow a flashlight, we'll check on Diamond and Prince on our way home."

"Do you think she would have delivered Prince on her own?" Katy asked as we started down the dirt road.

"Probably not. He's huge," I said. "Safe to say you saved his life, sweetie."

We reached the corner of the heifer pasture, killed the engine, and quietly stepped out of the car. Katy shined the flashlight across the fence. A newborn calf stood on four wobbly legs and shivered while his mother licked at him furiously. Then ever so gently, she nudged him with her nose, closer, until he latched on and began to nurse.

"I never get tired of this picture," Katy whispered. "It's such a gentle reminder of how sweet life is." She sighed. "I think maybe I'm ready for one of my own. What do you think?"

"What? You want a calf," I exclaimed.

"I'm serious, sweetie." She stared into my eyes. "I think we're ready for a baby."

I was caught completely by surprise. "Uh . . . well, maybe you're right." I wrapped my arms around her and held her tightly.

"Let's go home and . . . talk about it, or . . . something."

9 – Time for a Baby?

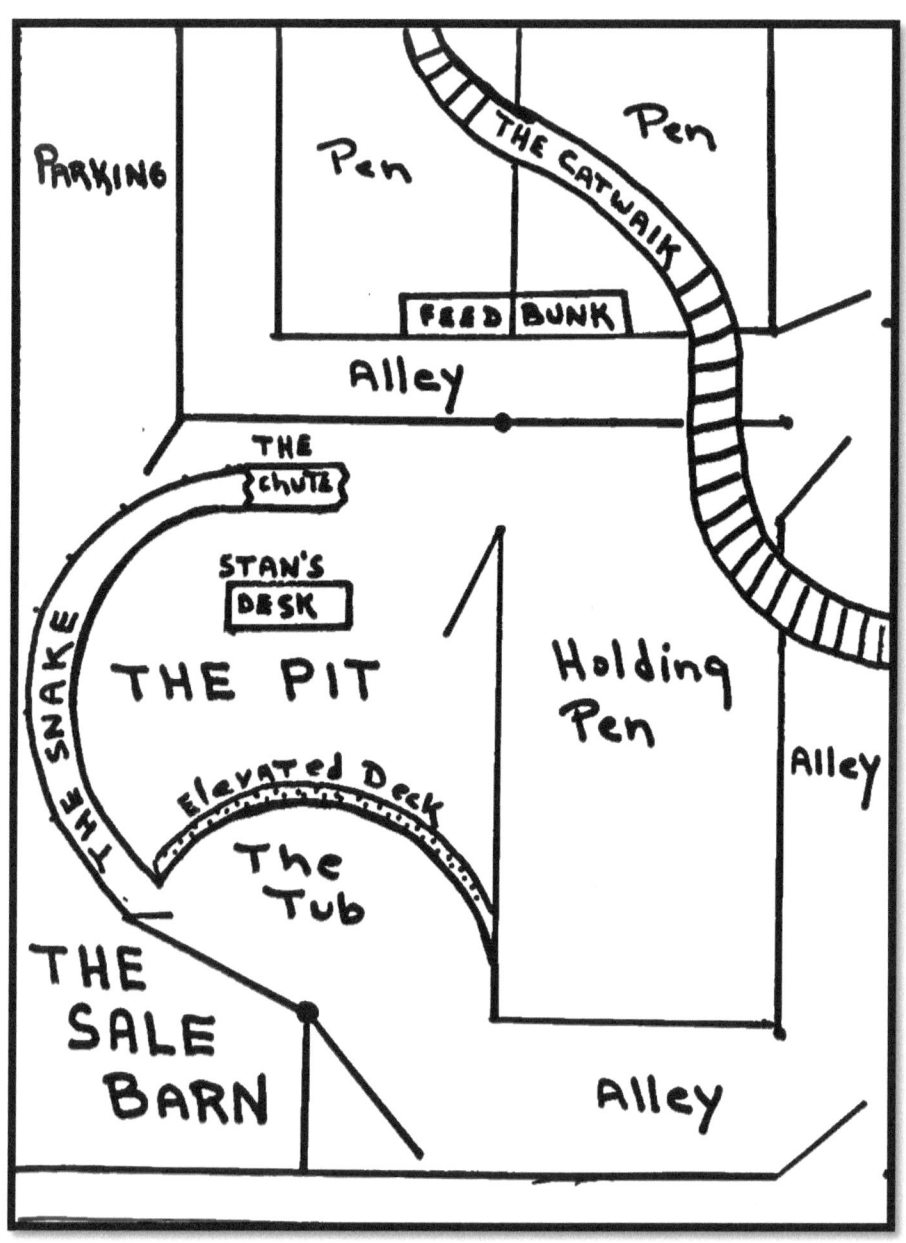

Chapter 10
THE DEVIL IN THE SALE BARN

It was noon when I drove in the front gate. A cloud of dust hung over the yard as the cowboys on horseback unloaded the cattle-filled trailers one after another. The long line of trailers was a good indication that it was going to be a long and busy day.

The day Mike and I decided to provide our services to the sale barn was the start of fourteen long years of working on alternate Sundays. The sale barn, a livestock auction, held a sale every Monday, which meant that preparations for the sale had to be finished on Sunday.

Every Monday morning, ranchers and cattle brokers from all over the state, some selling cattle, others buying, gathered and participated in the ancient art of bartering. The Roswell sale barn held the largest sales of any livestock auction in the state, often selling over two thousand cows, bulls, and calves in a day.

The yard was several acres of land covered by a honeycomb of ten-by-ten-foot steel pens, each with its own gate, water trough, and feed bunk. Groups of pens were separated by a series of alleys which the cowboys used to sort and pen cattle.

I parked close to the work site and slipped into my coveralls. I noticed Denny, the yard foreman, on the catwalk—an elevated, narrow walkway ten feet above the ground. It was a steel-framed structure with a wooden plank floor and metal pipe handrails. The catwalk serpentined back and forth across the entire yard and gave Denny a vantage point from which he supervised all that transpired below.

In the center of the yard was *the pit.* It wasn't really a pit, but rather the area where all cattle were processed the day before the sale. The pit had three sections—*the tub, the snake,* and *the chute.* The *tub* was a circular holding pen with solid metal sides which held up to thirty head of cattle at a time. Cattle were led from their pens down a series of alleys to the back side of the tub. Then a solid metal gate pivoted and closed behind them. At the front end of the *tub* was a gate that led to the *snake,* a fifty-foot narrow channel that extended and arched to the right, just wide enough to keep cattle moving in a single file as they headed to the *chute*—a heavy metal cage where they were processed one at a time. The *chute* had twin gates that opened and closed like a pair of scissors at the front and back ends. As a cow entered the chute, the back gates closed behind her and prevented her from backing out. The front gates closed on her neck, and the sides of the chute squeezed like bookends to safely restrain the cow. Everything was controlled by a small electric motor and three hydraulic levers, attached to the side of the chute.

The day before the sale, every animal to be sold passed through the pit. Each cow, bull or calf had a paper tag with an identification number glued to its side. All bulls and cows were required to have

10 – The Devil in the Sale Barn

blood drawn and tested for Brucellosis, a contagious and devastating disease. Most cows were pregnancy-tested. Today, that was my job.

The pit crew consisted of Stan, Bob, and either my partner or me. Stan identified and cataloged every animal that passed through the chute. He made sure the cowboys kept the tub full and returned cattle to their proper pen after they passed through the chute.

Stan was five feet six inches tall, wore a mustache, cowboy boots, and a cowboy hat. He was a religious man with a heart of gold and a serious fear of the devil. He was good at his job, but he talked too much.

In contrast to Stan, Bob was a shy and quiet man, lanky, with a good sense of humor. He enjoyed his work and seldom raised his voice, except when Stan talked too much. Bob was the "bleeder". His job was to draw blood for Brucellosis testing. As a cow or bull moved through the snake, Bob raised its tail with his left hand. His right hand held a blood tube and an attached needle which he injected into a vein under the tail. He collected two milliliters of blood, stored the numbered tube in a safe container, grabbed the next tube, and went on to the next cow. In all my years of practice, I never saw anyone more skilled at bleeding a cow on the run.

My job was to operate the chute and pregnancy-test the cows, a procedure not accomplished by analyzing blood, but rather by feel. I wore a plastic glove that covered the skin from my fingers up to my underarm. I inserted my entire arm up the cow's rectum and searched for a baby in the uterus, which is located directly beneath the colon. A two-month-old baby is the size of a golf ball, four-month-old, the size of a cat, six-month old, the size of a large dog. It was a filthy way of determining pregnancy, but at the time, it was still the fastest and most accurate.

The three of us were great buddies. We respected and more importantly, protected each other. We worked in what was by far, the most dangerous spot in the yard, a confined trap bordered on three sides by the tub, snake, and chute. But as long as I had Stan and Bob by my side, I felt relatively safe.

I walked into the pit and found Bob busy as he numbered his blood tubes and arranged them in groups of a hundred. Stan leafed through a stack of papers two inches thick, turned one page after another with unusual intensity.

"Afternoon. How are you guys today?" I asked with as much enthusiasm as I could. Sunday afternoon at the sale barn was not one of my favorite pastimes.

"Good to see you, Jim," Bob answered with his usual big smile and kind voice.

Stan said nothing. He shuffled through his paperwork as though he had lost something important. I looked at Bob who shrugged his shoulders.

"So, what's up Stan?" I broke his silence.

"Oh, hi, Jim." He looked at me as if I had just arrived.

"Listen, guys, we need to be extra careful today," Stan said.

"What's the occasion, Stan?" Bob asked.

"Did you guys see the new moon last night?" Stan asked, with fear in his voice.

10 – The Devil in the Sale Barn

"Can't say I did," Bob said. "Tell me about it."

"It was cradling a red glow. That red glow was the devil." Stan's hands trembled.

I was amused and Bob coughed loudly to disguise his laughter, but Stan wasn't joking. He was scared.

Stan wiped the sweat off his brow. "He's here, boys, hiding somewhere in the yard. He's here to make life miserable for us, so watch out," he warned.

"Stanley, I've got some garlic in my pickup you can wrap around your neck," Bob said and chuckled.

"Not funny, Bob!"

The conversation was entertaining, but we had a lot of work to do. "Well, sounds like we're in for a helluva day," I said as I slipped the plastic glove over my left hand and up my arm. "Are we ready to go?"

The cowboys pushed the first load of cows down the alley. Then I noticed a young, redheaded boy with a face full of freckles and a mouth full of braces. He stood on a narrow grate that was attached to the outside of the tub and allowed him to oversee the cows as they ran down the alley toward him.

"Who's the kid, Stan?" I asked. And, what's he doing down here where he has no business being, I wondered.

"That's Tiger. He's our *hot shot* man today," Stan said.

"You've gotta be kidding! What is he, maybe thirteen?" I exclaimed.

"I don't know," Stan replied. "He's Denny's nephew. Don't think he's had much experience with a hot shot."

The *hot shot* was our cattle prod, an instrument used to encourage cattle to keep moving forward when they would rather back up. The average battery-operated model delivers a low-level shock. Our hot shot was a little more sophisticated and a lot more dangerous. It was a wooden cane with a copper tip—a perfect conductor—attached to an overhanging insulated electrical cable which was hard-wired to the yard's electrical system. The prod delivered 110 volts to anything it touched. The worker who operated this near-lethal weapon, usually a yard hand who possessed few skills and lacked the capacity for abstract thinking, was randomly selected each week by Denny. Once the cattle were confined in the tub, the *hot shot* man's job was to keep them moving through the snake. Today, that job belonged to a snot-nosed kid—Tiger!

"Wonderful," I said and shook my head. "We really are in for a helluva day."

"Hey, Tiger, you know how to handle one of these?" I handed him the cane.

"You bet, Doc. I gotcha covered." He grabbed the cane by the handle and shook it like a warrior going into battle. God help us, I thought.

"Remember one thing, Tiger. A little bit of fire from that hot shot goes a long way. The more you use it, the more pissed off your cows will get. We don't need these cows pissed off any more than they already are. Understood?" I asked, expecting a response.

He answered with a *not really* look and nodded.

"Everybody ready," I yelled. I flipped the switch to the chute. The sound of cattle crowding into the tub was instantly drowned out by the whining of the electric motor. I made one last check with Tiger and, reluctantly, turned on the switch to the hot shot.

"You're hot now, Tiger! Be careful," I warned.

The cows moved into the snake and Bob drew his first blood sample. The first cow ran into the chute and I immediately closed the back gate. I caught her head with the front gate and squeezed the sides. I lowered a side panel on the chute, moved in behind the cow, inserted my hand deep into her rectum, found the uterus, and felt a calf. "She's pregnant, Stan—five months."

"Gotcha, Jim," he answered and noted it on his paper. Stan backtagged her and clipped a metal identification tag to her right ear. I made a final check to make sure everybody was clear and released the cow. She ran out of the chute as the next cow worked her way through the snake.

When the last cow of the bunch exited the chute, Stan chased her into the holding pen and closed a wide gate behind her. The gate had a spring-loaded bolt and it locked automatically when it slammed shut. With the cows safely separated from the pit, the cowboys moved them back to their original pen as the next group of cattle crowded into the tub.

We processed the first hundred cows in just over an hour. All was well, except for Tiger, who became more and more liberal with the use of the hot shot. Repeated reminders from Bob and me to back off began to fall on deaf ears.

We struggled with a group of *Tiger-striped* cows, a notoriously ill-tempered Hereford/Brahman cross. Tiger was unable to get the last cow into the snake. Repeated shocks with the hot shot did little more than add to her anger. When she finally ran into the snake, she was mad. I managed to catch her and we went to work. Bob bled her, I pregnancy-tested her, and Stan had her tagged, all in the span of thirty seconds.

"Turn her loose, Jim," Stan yelled. The front gate opened, the cow flew out of the chute, hit the ground, spun 180 degrees, and lowered her head. She was coming after us. Bob and I immediately dove into the empty snake, the safest spot we could find. The kid jumped into the tub. Stan wasn't quite fast enough. The only thing that separated him from the onrushing fury was his table. She hit it at full speed and lifted it up and over his head. Stan threw himself on the ground as she raced over the top of him kicking and bucking the whole way. She ran around the entire circle of the pit, scattered Bob's blood tubes and Stan's papers everywhere. Her quest for revenge satisfied, she gave a final snort and trotted out of the pit. Stan struggled to his feet, ran behind her and swung the gate to the holding pen.

"Didn't I tell you guys he was here," Stan said as he walked back to the pit, limping and out of breath.

"What are you talking about, Stan?" Bob was also catching his breath.

"The devil, Bob. The devil is in that cow."

"Shut up, Stan," Bob yelled, his brow furrowed. "There's no damn devil in that cow. She's just a pissed off cow!"

"Tiger! I want you to settle down with that hot shot or I'm going to shove it up your ass, you understand," Bob yelled angrily.

We took a break while Bob gathered his scattered blood tubes. Miraculously, none were damaged. Stan picked up papers. Tiger was a bit shaken as well by the vengeful cow and agreed to put the hot shot down for a while.

The following groups of cows were much easier to work and the next half hour was uneventful. Then an older and more stubborn cow entered the snake and stopped. She held up the line. Bob slapped her on the back, but she didn't budge. Against his better judgment, Bob called for the kid.

"Tiger. I need a little help over here." Tiger was given the green light and he sprang into action.

"Coming, Bob," he said with a new boost of confidence. He picked up the hot shot and ran directly toward the old cow. Then we heard the familiar *ZZZAP!* The cane contacted the cow and she lunged forward into the chute. With unbridled enthusiasm, Tiger turned to run back to the tub, swinging the hot shot wildly in the air. We heard the *ZZZAP* for the second time. The prod caught the tip of Bob's ear. It was only a slight touch, but the 110 volts was more than enough to drop Bob to his knees. It took us a moment before we realized what had happened. Tiger never did figure out what he had done.

When Bob finally came to his senses, he whispered to Stan, "Get rid of that little shit before I kill him."

All of us saw the look in Stan's eyes—that devil thing again.

"Shut up, Stan," Bob said before Stan could utter a word. "Let's go to work."

I bled the rest of the group for Bob while he rested and drank a Dr. Pepper. It happened that Denny was on the catwalk directly above the pit at the exact time of the incident and saw the whole thing. He whistled and gestured for Tiger to join him on the catwalk. That was the last we saw of the boy.

Bob recovered and we processed the next few sets of cows with amazing speed. Denny asked Kim, one of the best cowboys in the yard, to take over for Tiger. Kim knew how to work cows. He never touched the hot shot. Instead, he used a quiet but firm voice command and a slap on the back to persuade the cows to enter the snake.

Four o'clock arrived and it was time to feed the livestock. We decided to take a short break. Denny had an old flat-bed truck that the feeding crew stacked with hay. The bales were stacked high over the cab of the truck to limit the return trips to the hay barn for another load. The feeding crew was a two-man operation. One drove the truck through the alleys between pens while the other stood on top of the haystack and tossed bales into the feed bunks of each pen. Occasionally, the truck had to cross under the catwalk.

Because of the small clearance between the top of the haystack and the underside of the catwalk, the feeder had to hop off the haystack and onto the catwalk, then hop back onto the moving haystack as the truck passed underneath. It was a simple procedure understood by most of the workers in the yard. Eventually, the stack got low enough to allow for ducking under the catwalk.

10 – The Devil in the Sale Barn

We waited for the cowboys to bring more cattle. The feed truck rolled up the alley next to the pit, made a hard left turn and proceeded toward an intersection with the catwalk. Today, the man on top of the stack was Junior, a young African American kid with a big Afro hairdo and a body no bigger around than a pencil. Junior was usually assigned to the clean-up crew and had never been on the feeding crew. The truck carried a full load. Junior wore a sleeveless t-shirt and baggy pants and he danced on top of the stack as though he were performing for his fans on the big stage. He suddenly became aware of the approaching catwalk. He stopped dancing and looked around, unsure of what to do. Everyone saw the situation unfold, but nobody gave it much thought, as we assumed common sense would provide the obvious solution to Junior's puzzle.

"Surely, he's not going . . ." Before Stan finished his sentence, he saw the nightmare unfold. "No, you idiot!" he yelled.

Junior decided to lay flat on his back on top of the haystack. Apparently, he felt confident that his skinny body would clear the catwalk.

"He's not going to make it," Bob said. He whistled as loudly and as high-pitched as he could, to get the drivers' attention. "Stop, stop!" he shouted. It was too late.

Junior was under the catwalk. He would have been okay were it not for the sharp ends of the wires that tied the wooden planks to the frame. The blood-curdling scream echoed throughout the yard as the wires ripped through his clothes and the skin on his legs and chest like a knife through butter.

Stan reached the truck and banged on the hood. *"Back up, back up!"* he shouted. The driver realized that Junior was in trouble. He slammed on the brake, shifted the truck into reverse, and backed out from under the catwalk.

We lowered Junior from the haystack. I ran to my truck and retrieved bandage material. We gently wrapped junior's chest and legs and did what we could to distract him from the pain while we waited for the ambulance. It was quickly evident to all of us that Stan had saved Junior's face and possibly his life.

Stan turned to Bob and me with a stern look on his face. "You believe me now?"

"Shut up, Stan," Bob answered. "We've got another hundred cows to do before we can get the hell out of here. Let's just get it done, okay?"

"Okay, Bob, but I've got a bad feeling he's not done with us yet," Stan said. Bob shook his head. It was now after five and the sun was setting. The lights in the yard came on and made the dust in the air look like a foggy scene out of a horror movie. We worked for an hour without any incident.

Denny appeared on the catwalk overlooking the pit. "Stan! We have one more bunch—twenty-five cows."

I saw the relief on Stan's face. Twenty-five more cows and he could slip out of this hell trap and away from the grip of the devil. The Hereford cows in the tub were big, muscular, and passive. They filed into the snake like obedient pets. Stan counted them down one at a time and then the last cow of the day was in the chute. Bob bled her, I

10 – The Devil in the Sale Barn

pregnancy-tested her, and Stan tagged her. Then he broke into a joyful dance around the pit as if he had just won the lottery.

"Turn her loose, Jim," he yelled.

I opened the front gate of the chute and the cow trotted out toward the holding pen as Stan walked behind her.

"Ha! We did it Jim! We cheated the devil!" Stan cried out in glee. He grabbed the gate to the holding pen and swung it as hard as he could. The latch was within inches of locking when it hit the easy-natured cow at the base of her tail. Instinctively, she threw her butt up in the air, kicked with both back feet, and launched the gate like a cannon ball.

Stan never saw it coming. The top rail hit him right above his eyes and shot him into the air like a rag doll. He landed hard on the ground and was motionless. I thought he might be dead. Bob would later admit that he was certain of it. He was unconscious for what seemed an eternity, but he finally recovered, and Bob took him to the hospital. He later reported that on the way there, Stan mumbled over and over again, 'The sonofabitch got me after all.' This time, Bob decided to just let it go.

Later that night, I visited Stan and Junior in the emergency room. Junior received seventy-five stitches in his chest and legs. Stan got an ice pack on his forehead.

"He tried his best to kill me, Jim," Stan said as he looked at me through two black eyes.

Somewhere off in the distance, at home, sitting in his favorite chair drinking a beer, I could hear Bob's voice—"Shut up, Stan!"

MY FRIENDS WALK BAREFOOT

Chapter 11

JAY MEETS CARRIE

On May 11, 1985, Katy's and my life changed forever. John Thomas came into our lives. We named our first-born son after his grandfather and called him JT. He became the focal point of our days and nights and we wanted to spend every waking moment with our baby boy. Yet, Katy and I were determined not to let our little bundle of joy interfere with our relationship with our friends.

Jay and Dana were not just friends, they were family. For four years, we had laughed together, cried together, and learned that we could depend on each other at any time and in any circumstance. As babies always do, they grow quickly, and so do their demands. Those wonderful nights, enhanced by great food, margaritas, beer, and wine, previously unencumbered by such details as a baby, were soon cut short by our need to get home and put our son to bed. The weekend evenings with our friends became few and far between.

For a while, we were able to balance what we once had with what we now had, but eventually, things changed. We found new friends, as did Jay and Dana. That common thread that for years, had held us together tightly, gradually unraveled.

Because we seldom saw them, we were unaware of a new development in their relationship. Dana graduated from nursing school and decided that being a rancher's wife was not what she wanted out of life. In time, they divorced and Dana was gone.

It was a tough time for Jay. Katy and I did what we could to be supportive. We invited him to our house for supper on occasion, but the ranch was now his life and he had little time to spare.

One Saturday morning, I received an unexpected call. "Jim, it's Jay. Let's go plinkin." 'Plinkin' was Jay's term for target shooting. On the south side of his ranch, Jay had a gravel pit with huge dirt barriers that provided the perfect backstop for safe shooting of any weapon.

"Sounds great. I'll be there in half an hour," I said.

Targets were set. Jay leaned over the hood of his truck, looked through the scope attached to his new 8mm Mauser, took a deep breath, and whispered, "Jim, I met a girl last weekend." He squeezed the trigger. The blast echoed through the pit. He looked at me with a child-like grin.

I was astonished and curious. "Oh, yeah? So, are you gonna tell me more or do I have to beat it out of you with a stick?" I laughed, still mystified, but excited for Jay. It had been close to a year since Dana had left and he had lived alone during those months, not an easy task for a man as gregarious as Jay.

"My sister, Sharon, has been bugging me about coming to Dallas," he said. "So, I flew down for the weekend. She introduced me to a friend. Her name is Carrie. I know what you're thinking. It's just a sexual thing, right? Well, you know what? This girl's special."

11 – Jay Meets Carrie

"So, when do we get to meet her?" I asked with a broad smile.

"Soon. She's a pharmaceutical rep., shorter than I am, red hair, pretty smile, a bundle of energy. She has a couple weeks of vacation. Gonna come out and spend some time with me," Jay said, attempting to disguise a sheepish smile.

Carrie flew out for a visit and fell in love with Jay and the ranch. She quit her job in Dallas, decided to stay, and married Jay.

The years passed. It wasn't just like old times, but then why should it be. We were all older. Katy and I now had two boys. Jay was principal owner of the ranch. And yet, somehow, I felt like I had my buddy back. As for Carrie, well, everybody loved Carrie. She thrived at being a ranch hand and quickly learned the particulars of the business—a huge advantage for Jay. Once again, we became great friends.

Carrie convinced Jay that there was a better way to maximize profit in ranching. She researched and compiled accurate records on each individual cow—her age, her physical condition, and whether she had raised a calf the previous year. She also questioned whether leasing the farmland to the neighbor, a guy who appeared to live like the richest man in town, was a good idea. Perhaps Jay should not renew the leases, invest in farm equipment, and reap the rewards of farming himself. With each passing year, Carrie developed a greater sense of how things should be done. Her business recommendations, in time, helped Jay become a more successful farmer-rancher.

Time seems to change the need for certain pleasures, but some pleasures manage to escape time. Jay still loved to party. It was the summer of 1997 when Jay and Carrie decided to have a 4th of July party to celebrate the birth of our nation with a hundred of their closest friends.

Eddie owned the local fireworks manufacturing company. Jay had allowed Eddie to hunt on the ranch and in appreciation, Eddie delivered a truckload of boxes filled with fireworks that made the city's display look like a kiddy sparkler show.

The assortment included sparklers for the kids, smoke bombs, firecrackers, bottle rockets, helicopters, whistlers, four- and six-inch mortars that flew hundreds of feet into the air and exploded into huge visual extravaganzas, and for the grand finale, 250,000 roman candles. When I first heard the number, I didn't believe it, but when we counted the number of candles per box and the number of boxes, there were indeed, 250,000 roman candles, each capable of shooting 10 flaming balls into the air.

Jay and I, along with my co-worker, Santiago, cooked a pig, a whole pig, from scratch, Mexican style—*carnitas, chicharrones, and carne adobada.* As usual, Jay had plenty of beer.

With unwavering energy, Carrie hustled from the garage to the front lawn and set up tables and chairs. She prepared a banquet the likes of which most people would have had catered. Carrie personally greeted her arriving guests, organized games for the kids to play, and made sure their faces were lathered with sunscreen and that they were well hydrated.

Jay and I strategically placed the fireworks in a dry field in front of the ranch headquarters. The plan was to light the smaller stuff first,

11 – Jay Meets Carrie

move on to the big mortars, and finish with the roman candles, still in boxes which were set up in a long straight line directly in front of, and at a not-so-safe distance from where the viewing crowd would be seated.

At sunset, Carrie called for everyone to gather their lawn chairs in preparation for the grand event. Her face beamed with pride as she read a brief history of the ranch. Jay looked on, his chest held high. I had never seen him so happy.

By show time, Jay and I had consumed enough beer to slightly, or perhaps more than slightly, dull the senses. Jay had the entire show choreographed in his mind—start slow, let it build up, and finish with a grand finale that will be remembered for years.

Jay and I lit the first fuses. Two bottle rockets flew into the air in perfect harmony. Then came the unexpected. The first of the two rockets landed directly in the middle of the fuses that lit the mortars and set off a spectacular chain reaction. Instead of the mortars exploding one after another, five exploded simultaneously, then ten, then twenty. The crowd cheered, unaware that the plan had gone completely wrong.

The second bottle rocket took a bit longer before it landed directly in the center of the line of roman candles. The ensuing fire spread in both directions down the row of boxes. Flaming balls began to fly. At first, a few, then more and more, and more. They flew vertically, horizontally, and in every direction. The inebriated section of the crowd yelled for more. The more sober ran for cover. In retrospect, Jay and I were lucky to get out alive.

Within five minutes, Jay and Carrie's ranch became a fireworks display like never before seen in the entire state of New Mexico. A local deputy sheriff who was patrolling miles away became alarmed when he saw the distant glow and drove at full speed toward the ranch. He arrived, stepped out of his car, and stood silent, in awe of the spectacular show. Then he quietly got back in his car and left. The sky was lit up for the next hour and the remains burned for the rest of the night. The event was talked about for years by those lucky to have witnessed the spectacular debacle.

Summer gave way to fall. November was usually the month that Jay gathered his pastures, weaned and vaccinated his calves, and called me to pregnancy-test his cows. The crew consisted of Santiago and me along with Jay and two or three of his cowboys.

A cold front had moved in the night before. The morning was extremely cold. A stiff wind welcomed Santiago and me as we stepped out of my pickup and quickly numbed the tips of our ears and noses. The cowboys had separated cows from their calves and positioned the cows in a pen that led to the chute where I was to pregnancy-test them one at a time. Everyone wore arctic gear, heavy jackets with hoodies and gloves.

I shook hands with Jay. "You sure know how to pick 'em," I said, referring to his choice to pregnancy-test cows on the lousiest day we had seen all year.

"Hey, you know what I always say. Nothing you and I do together ever comes easy," he said with a big smile. "Why break with tradition?"

11 – Jay Meets Carrie

From over Jay's shoulder, I heard a familiar voice. "Good morning, Jim."

The face was partially covered by the thick hood of a jacket, but the smile was unmistakable. "Carrie?"

"How are you this fine morning?" she asked.

"What the hell are you doing here?" I was surprised at first and then impressed by the site of Carrie, eager to contribute in the midst of a real shitty day.

"Oh, didn't Jay tell you?" she asked, her lips trembling from the cold. "I'm in charge today."

It took me a minute to realize what a subtle, yet very effective spanking I had just been given. I smiled. "Of course you are, Boss. What do you say we get started so we can get out of this crappy weather?"

Santiago operated the chute. I pregnancy-tested the cows. Jay vaccinated and called out the cow's ear tag numbers to Carrie, who marked the numbers along with the rest of the data on her record sheet.

The first cow ran into the chute and we went to work. With a plastic glove that covered my left hand and reached up to my shoulder, I thrust my arm into the cow's rectum, found her uterus directly below the colon, and felt the calf inside. "She's six months pregnant, Carrie," I yelled.

"Thanks, Jim," she said and recorded the information on a sheet of paper.

By mid-morning, we had run nearly a hundred cows through the chute. The weather conditions declined by the hour. It began to sleet and the wind chill factor made the temperature feel as if in the teens. Carrie's paperwork was wet and her pens wouldn't write. Eventually she was forced to stuff everything inside her jacket against her chest.

"Carrie, maybe you'd better go to the house. We'll finish this," Jay said.

"Trying to get rid of me, are you? I don't think so. Who's going to keep these records straight—you?" Carrie replied. Jay said nothing and the miserable process continued.

The cowboys worked methodically and kept the cows filing into the chute. Jay owned a manual chute and without the aid of hydraulics, Santiago's arm and shoulder muscles fatigued under the stress of squeezing and releasing each cow from the massive metal cage. I glanced at Carrie. Her hands trembled and her lips quivered from the cold.

One of the cowboys yelled, "Ten more cows, ya'll. Git 'er done." The next cow ran into the chute. Santiago caught and squeezed her.

I walked into the chute from behind ready to pregnancy-test her when I heard Jay yell, "Whoa! Wait a minute, Jim. Don't bother with her. She's old. We'll sell her."

"What do you mean, we'll sell her?" Carrie asked as I walked out from behind the chute.

"She's old, Carrie. She needs to be somebody else's problem."

"What if she's pregnant?"

I sensed a battle brewing.

"I could care less. She's a grandma. She needs to go to town," Jay exclaimed.

11 – Jay Meets Carrie

"I'd like for Jim to pregnancy-test her," she said with conviction.

Jay looked at me and sighed. His frustration was well noted. "Okay! Check her, Jim."

It was the biggest calf I had felt all day. "She'll have this calf within a month," I said, confidently.

"Maybe she needs to stay. What do you think, Jim?" Carrie asked, hoping for my support. "Should we keep her?"

I looked at Carrie, then at Jay and then, back at Carrie. I was smart enough to know, as Jay was, that even though she was pregnant and due to deliver soon, at her age, this cow may be incapable of raising her calf. I tried to decide which side of this bread was better buttered and finally said, "Uh, well, I suppose . . . Uh, yeah, I suppose she might make it another year. Carrie smiled. I read Jay's lips.

"You traitor!" Jay mouthed, disgusted with losing the debate.

"She's lost her ear tag, Carrie," Jay yelled. "You need to give her another one."

Carrie scrambled to the toolbox and found a new ear tag and the pliers necessary to pin it to the cow's ear. She leaned directly above the cow's head and pinched the pliers, penetrating the ear with a sharp fastener that attached the new tag. Without warning, the cow threw her head up and connected squarely with Carrie's chest and chin. Carrie flew into the air and landed on the ground, flat on her back.

We were all stunned. Jay was closest. He ran to her and threw himself to his knees. "Are you okay?"

Carrie lay on her back, eyes closed. "I'm okay. Just give me a minute." We all stood perfectly still, amazed that she was conscious, much less talking. After a couple of deep breaths, she sat up, rubbed her chin, and slowly rose to her feet. She walked over to the old lady, careful to stay out of head butt range, and looked the cow straight in the eye. "You ever pull a stunt like that again, I just might let him sell you," she warned.

"Okay, guys. Throw them some hay and let's get the hell outta here," Jay yelled to his crew as the last cow left the chute. A tough day was finally over.

That evening, Katy and the boys cuddled on the couch under a wool blanket in front of a roaring fire as I walked through the front door.

"Papa's home, boys. Come join us, sweetie," Katy said.

I hadn't showered and my face and hands still carried a layer of dust lightly sprinkled with specks of dried cow manure. I removed my jacket, boots, and socks and sat on the tile floor in front of the fireplace.

"Oh, this feels good," I said.

"Well, how did it go?" Katy asked.

"We froze our butts off," I replied. I rubbed my hands together briskly. "Aside from that, it was a great day. Nobody got hurt—well almost, but not bad."

"How did the cows do?" she asked.

"We had over ninety percent pregnant."

"Wow! That's great. I'll bet Jay was thrilled."

"It was kinda hard to know how anyone was feeling. The cold had all of us sort of numbed. I'm sure Jay was happy." I paused for a moment. "So was the new boss."

"New boss?" Katy cocked her head to one side and raised an eyebrow. "Carrie was there?" she asked.

"Yup. She ran the whole show," I said. "Did a helluva good job, too."

"Wow! Well, it's about time somebody kept Jay in line," Katy said, with a devilish smirk on her face. Then that smirk softened to a genuine smile. "I'm really happy for him."

I rested my feet on the hearth in front of the fire. Blood slowly filtered its way back into my frozen toes. I lay back and sighed. "Yeah. Me too, sweetie. Me too." I closed my eyes and reflected on events that had changed my life, and the special gifts that had not changed—the warmth of a fire on a cold winter's night, the love of my family, and the joy of having a great friend.

MY FRIENDS WALK BAREFOOT

Chapter 12
HERSHEY

His name was Luke Greenfield. He was in his mid-thirties, six feet tall with long blonde hair and blue eyes. Luke was usually unshaven and wore tattered clothes that looked like they had been slept in for weeks. He was a gentle man, kind and quiet, but he never left my office without a genuine handshake and a sincere, "Thanks, Doc. I sure do appreciate you." He struggled to disguise the tremor in his hands, but he couldn't hide the uncontrollable blinking of his eyes. He spoke with a touch of sadness.

Luke had a pair of Bull Terriers, Butkus and Ruby. The Bull Terrier breed is a forty-five to fifty-pound mass of muscle with short hair, a large egg-shaped head, small eyes, short erect ears, a powerful jaw, and a sweet personality. Ruby had raised several litters of puppies sired by Butkus and because both dogs had such great looks and wonderful dispositions, Ruby's pups were in huge demand.

Luke never told me how much money he got for his pups, but it was clear that he was very particular about who would be allowed to buy one. "None of my pups will ever be trained to fight," he once told me. "Anyone who gets a pup from me needs to treat him like a first-born kid." He interviewed all prospective buyers and if they didn't meet his high standards, they didn't get a pup—at any price.

One morning, I had the pleasure of giving the first vaccinations to Ruby's most recent litter—five females and one male. The females were predominantly white with random brown and black splotches painted across their faces, bodies, and feet. The male, the biggest of the litter by far, looked like he had been dipped in a vat of milk chocolate. Luke called him Hershey. I knew from the day I first saw him, this pup would never be sold. Luke paid his bill with cash, as usual. He never offered to tell me what he did for a living and I didn't ask.

It was a beautiful evening. Katy read a bedtime story to the boys as I watched pink clouds turn bright orange and then crimson, as dusk turned to darkness. Perfect evenings were often interrupted when I was on call. Tonight was no different. My pager rang. The message read, *Call Mr. Greenfield, A.S.A.P. Dog in trouble.* I dialed the number.

"Doc! It's Hershey. I don't know what's going on. He was fine a little while ago, but he's freaking out. I think he's dying. Can you meet me?" I sensed panic in his voice.

I grabbed keys off the kitchen counter and peeked in on Katy and the boys. "Gotta go. I'll be back soon." So many of the emergency calls I answered were silly overreactions that could easily wait until the next day, but something told me this was not one of those calls.

As I drove up, Luke paced back and forth at the front door of the hospital with Hershey cradled in his arms.

"Follow me," I said. I unlocked the door. We hurried through the reception area straight to the patient treatment room. I heard Hershey's mournful cries, not a sound of pain, just mournful, I thought.

"Let me have him, Luke." He gripped his pup tightly. His hands trembled. "It's okay, Luke. I've got him. Let's lay him down on the table," I said as my hand gently touched his shoulder. Slowly, he released Hershey and allowed me to examine him. The pup's pupils were both widely dilated and all four legs paddled aimlessly. His head swayed back and forth as if he were trying unsuccessfully to focus on a given spot.

"Is there a chance he's been hurt, Luke?" I asked.

"No way, Doc. He's been with me all day."

"Any vomiting or diarrhea?"

"No, sir. He was fine an hour ago. I was watching TV when I heard something weird. I found him in the bedroom like this and called you right away."

Hershey's symptoms didn't seem to fit what I expected of either a poison or trauma case. Most of the poisons he might have ingested should cause vomiting, diarrhea, muscle tremors, or seizures. Luke seemed certain there had been no head injury. The pup moaned and looked about as if in a dream.

"What do you think?" Luke asked as he tried desperately to control his emotions.

"I'm not sure, but I think he's hallucinating."

"What do you mean?"

"I think he's trippin' out. Is there anything you can think of that he might have gotten into?" I asked with urgency.

"He's been in the house with me, Doc. The last of his five sisters went to her new home this afternoon so he's been kinda missing them, I guess. He was outside for a while just to pee, but I was right there with him," he said with assuredness.

"Tell you what we're going to do, Luke. You're going to hold onto him while I get a catheter in a vein. I really need your help on this," I insisted. "Passing out on me is not an option, okay?"

"I'm okay. I was in the infantry in 'Nam. Seen some pretty nasty stuff, Doc."

That was the first time he had ever mentioned anything to me about Vietnam. I could only imagine what horrific, life-changing events he must have witnessed.

Suddenly, it came to me. It all made sense. The military fatigue jacket that he wore with the shoulder patch identifying him as infantry, the nervous tremors, the melancholy. I had never heard of post-traumatic stress disorder, but I had suspected for some time that something had left Luke with scars much deeper than those visible on his hands and face.

I hadn't gone to Vietnam, but I had deep respect and empathy for all who had fought in that unpopular war. Many of the survivors were badly wounded, physically, mentally, or both. Worse, they returned home to anything but a hero's welcome. It was a travesty that made even the greatest of patriots, military and civilians, who had not been called to fight, consider themselves lucky.

12 - Hershey

I shaved the hair from one of Hershey's front legs and applied a tourniquet just above his elbow exposing the cephalic vein. "Ready? Hold him as still as you can." The twenty-two-gauge needle guided its indwelling catheter easily into the vein. I was concerned that the blood flowing back through the catheter might bother Luke, but he was steady. I removed the tourniquet, capped the catheter, and taped it to the leg. Luke watched as I connected the line that would drip the intravenous solution into Hershey's blood stream and force his kidneys to flush whatever it was that had a grip on him, out of his body. I administered ten milligrams of Valium into the IV line and within seconds, Hershey relaxed.

"Please tell me he's going to be all right," Luke said, his cheeks streaked with tears.

"We're halfway there, Luke. I have to give him something that's going to make him sick. I assume he's eaten something that's causing all this. He needs to vomit. This part gets unpleasant," I said. "I want you to go home and let me get to work."

"No! I'll stay and help you." His tone was strong and emphatic.

"Luke, I need you to go home and check on Butkus and Ruby. Call me if either of them is acting weird. Don't worry about Hershey," I said calmly. "I'll take good care of him. I promise. I expect him to be over this by morning." That was an overconfident assumption on my part, but he needed the reassurance. "I'll call you in the morning."

He considered my request for a long time, then he wiped the tears from his eyes and nodded. "Okay, Doc. Call me if there is any change."

"I will. Go get some sleep." I was pretty sure that wouldn't happen. With Luke out the door, I locked it and ran back to check on Hershey. He was relaxed, but awake.

I sprinkled ten milligrams of Apomorphine powder directly underneath Hershey's lower eyelid. It dissolved instantly, was absorbed into his blood stream, and the powerful stimulant directed his brain to induce vomiting. It took less than five minutes for effect. A minute later, the entire contents of his stomach lay on the table. It was mostly food, a few grass leaves, and three strange items.

I gathered them and washed them off in the sink, brown balloons, collapsed, but not empty. Each one was stuffed with something that felt mushy. One of the balloons had several holes in it. Hershey must have bitten into it before he swallowed it, I thought. With a scalpel blade, I sliced open the damaged balloon and exposed about a tablespoon of a dark sticky paste. I had never seen anything quite like it before, but I felt certain it was responsible for Hershey's wild *trip*.

I began to piece together a picture that I didn't like. I tried to ignore it, but it just wouldn't go away. How could this be? Was Luke a drug dealer? I was finding it hard to come up with another explanation and it hurt. I really liked this guy.

I threw the opened balloon into the trash along with the rest of the stomach contents, put the last two balloons in a plastic bag, and placed them in the refrigerator. The puppy's state of exhaustion combined with the effects of the Valium, allowed me to easily pass a tube through his mouth and into his stomach. With a large syringe, I delivered sixty milliliters of a gruel, a combination of water and activated charcoal. With any luck, it would bond to any remaining toxic substance in his intestines and prevent it from being absorbed into circulation. I cleaned him up, put him in a cage, checked his vitals, and covered him with a blanket. The intravenous fluids would run through his body and out by way his kidneys all night, purging his system. Time to go home.

I had quite a dilemma on my hands. What could I say to Luke tomorrow? Should I just ask him what the balloons were filled with? Maybe I'd get lucky and he would confess that Hershey had raided his private stash. What would my partner Mike suggest I should do, I wondered. Just as well he was on vacation. It was a good bet that Luke and I were both in for a sleepless night.

The next morning, I arrived at the office and found a healthy, happy puppy. He had chewed his IV drip line into tiny pieces, wagged his tail, and barked as if to say, *What's for breakfast. I'm hungry.* I fed him a small amount of soft food which he inhaled without chewing.

I called Luke with the good news. He cried so hard, he could hardly speak. "Thank you, Doc. When should I come get him?"

"We had better count on tomorrow, Luke. I'd like to keep an eye on him today," I said. I started to ask about the balloons, but stopped myself, hoping he would beat me to it.

"Tomorrow will be great," he said. "I have some stuff to take care of today, anyway. I'll try to get by this afternoon. If not, I'll see you tomorrow. Thanks again, Doc."

Neither of us mentioned the balloons. Why didn't I say something, I wondered. Was it fear of knowing the truth? Whatever the reason, it didn't change the fact that I needed to know what this stuff was.

I called Dan Carp, a client and good friend who worked for the local medical diagnostic lab. "Dan, I need a favor. I'd like you to look at something I came across last night. I'm hoping you can identify it." Without going into detail, I summarized the situation.

"Sure, Jim. Be glad to. Drop it by anytime," he said.

It was late afternoon before I was able to get to his office. The balloons were in a cardboard box wrapped with enough tape to plug the hole in the Titanic. The receptionist assured me that she would personally deliver the package to Dan.

The next morning, our receptionist, Roseann, met me as I came through the front door. "Dan Carp wants you to call him right away." I ran straight into my office and shut the door.

"Dan? It's Jim. What did you find out?"

"Your pup has very expensive taste, Jim. He swallowed a small fortune."

"What are you talking about? What the hell is that stuff?"

"Those balloons each contained about half an ounce of very high-grade hash."

"Hash? As in, hashish?"

"Yup," he answered with authority.

"I don't get it. This stuff doesn't look like pot, Dan."

"That's because it's not just ground up and dried. The flowers are processed into the concentrated paste that you sent me. The THC levels are a helluva lot higher," he continued. "Think of it this way, Jim. If marijuana is the grape juice of Cannabis, then hashish is the champagne."

"Wow. Thanks, Dan. I owe you one," I said, still stunned. "So, what did you do with the stuff?"

"Are you kidding? I smoked it! I saved a little bit to sprinkle on my breakfast cereal tomorrow. This is primo shit, man." He laughed. "What do you think I did with it? I packaged the whole thing up and sent it on to the police department."

"You did what!" I tried to disguise my shock.

"I sent it to the police. You *do* know this stuff is illegal, don't you, Jim?"

"Oh, sure, Dan. I guess I hadn't thought about it. Hey, thanks again." I hung up. Well, shit, I thought. Where do you go from here, smart guy? I massaged the temples of my aching head and walked to the treatment room. Andrew, the young man who kept our kennels clean, waited for me.

"How's Hershey?" I asked.

"He just had a bowel movement and passed these. I washed them up." He held up a paper towel with three more balloons.

I calmly took the balloons, put them in a plastic bag, placed the bag in the refrigerator, and smiled. "Thanks, Andrew." He looked at me suspiciously, but didn't ask anything.

It was just before noon when I finished the last surgery of the day. Roseann poked her head in the door. "Dr. Humphreys? There's a gentleman here to see you. He's not wearing a uniform, but he claims he's from the police department."

The shit had officially hit the fan. "Tell him I'll be with him in just a minute." I went to the bathroom, washed my hands and face several times, ran my fingers through my hair, and checked to see if anything was stuck between my teeth. When I couldn't find anything else to prolong the inevitable, I walked up front.

"Dr. Humphreys? I'm Detective Martinez," he said and extended his hand. "Can we talk in private?"

"Sure, come on back," I replied and shook his hand. As we walked to my office, Detective Martinez studied everything that hung on the walls—my diploma, my licenses, family pictures. He inspected each individual frame as if it possibly held potential clues to a murder.

"Have a seat, detective." I hoped he wouldn't see the sweat building on my forehead. After he had thoroughly examined all four walls, he sat down.

"I guess you know why I'm here," he said without smiling.

"Yup." That was all I could come up with. Then I remembered the last three balloons. "Excuse me, Detective. I'll be right back." I raced to the refrigerator, retrieved the last of the evidence, and was back in the office in a matter of seconds. "I think you may want these. The pup passed them this morning. They've been washed," I said and handed him the bag. He looked at it intensely as though he might find a valuable fingerprint on a balloon. I decided not to remind him that those balloons had been bathed in dog crap and washed in the sink.

"Doc, I need to know this guy's name," he said nonchalantly.

12 - *Hershey*

"His name is Hershey," I said. It was the first thing that came to mind.

"What?" He looked at me, confused.

"Hershey. His name is Hershey," I repeated.

"I'm not playing games, Doc. You know what I mean. I want to know who this dope peddler is." The tone of his voice was now serious.

"Mr. Martinez, would you explain to me what the deal is with stuffing hashish into balloons instead of plastic baggies?" I asked as I felt the first drop of sweat roll down my back.

He took a deep breath and decided to humor me. "He's probably taking the dope to the state penitentiary in Santa Fe. He either knows somebody on the inside or has a friend on the outside. You know they have visitation days at the pen. A family member is allowed to have a supervised picnic lunch with a convict. Did you notice that the balloons were all brown? Makes them less conspicuous," he continued. "The person on the outside sneaks the balloons to the person on the inside, who in turn, swallows them—when the guards aren't looking, of course. Eventually, those brown balloons come out the other end. Behind bars, they're worth ten times average street value." There was a long pause. "I need his name, Doc."

It was hard to look at him. My heart beat faster and my mind raced. What should I do? Just tell him. Why was I defending Luke? He was a drug dealer. Then again, if Mr. Martinez was right, he may not be pushing to local kids. What if he was? And if he wasn't, did that make what he was doing any less wrong? What if the guys whose habits he eased were also Vietnam veterans who shared his nightmares? Too many unanswered questions. The only thing I knew for sure was that Luke Greenfield loved his dogs like I loved my kids. That was going to have to be good enough for now. I looked Detective Martinez straight in the eyes. "I'm sorry, Detective. I can't do that."

He was startled at first, then he smiled and said, "Is this part of that doctor/client confidentiality bullshit you're pulling, Doc?"

"Something like that, I guess."

"You know I have the right to bring you down to the station for further questioning, don't you?"

Wow, I thought. Wakeup calls didn't get any better than this. My next telephone call to Katy would be from jail. I took my time, considered my options, and finally said, "Sorry. I can't do it." We both sat silent for a long time.

"Tell you what, Doc," he finally said. "I don't give a damn if this guy's selling drugs to cons. Hell, they deserve what they get. What I want, is to make sure he's not dealing locally. He could be pushing to our kids, you know," he said with a stern voice. "What if you were to tell me the general neighborhood he lives in—say, two to three blocks either way? I can put a patrol car in the area. If he's not dealing locally, there won't be any suspicious activity going on around his place." He sat back in his chair and waited for my reply. I was still uncomfortable with it, but decided the compromise was one I could live with.

"Okay," I said. I drew a map of the area that surrounded Luke's house, careful not to give any clues as to the actual address.

"Thanks, Doc," Detective Martinez said as he took the map and shook my hand.

"Uh, sir, is there . . . anything else you'll be needing from me? Are we okay?" I asked nervously.

"Don't worry, Doc. You're okay. Take care." He smiled, turned, and was gone.

The office closed at five thirty. It was just after five when Roseann caught me on my way to an exam room. "Mr. Greenfield is here to pick up Hershey."

"Put him in room three," I said.

I walked into the room with Hershey. As soon as Luke saw him, he broke into tears. Hershey recognized him immediately and barked with excitement. Luke lifted his pup gently from my arms and hugged him tightly. The more Luke cried, the faster Hershey licked the tears from his buddy's face.

I allowed a moment to enjoy the beauty of a relationship between a man and his dog. "We need to talk," I said. The smile on his face didn't fade. "How did he get the balloons, Luke?"

He stood perfectly still for a long time and stared at Hershey. Then he shook his head. "It was my fault, Doc. After I got through processing and weighing everything, I left the balloons in a box on a low shelf at the back of my closet." He kissed Hershey and the tears came once again. "The little shit is so curious. He gets into everything," he said with frustration. "It was stupid of me to leave it within his reach. I didn't even think about it again until the next morning when I found the box turned upside down and realized some balloons were missing. I should have told you yesterday when we talked, but by then, you had already saved his life. I was ashamed to admit to you that I had almost killed him."

I took off my glasses, peered through the dirty lenses, wiped them with a hand towel, took a deep breath, and slowly released it. "I had a visit from a detective today, Luke. I needed to know what the stuff was. If you and I had just talked about it yesterday morning, it might have saved us both a lot of grief. That was as much my fault as yours," I said as I shook my head. "Instead, I asked a friend to look at the balloons. The next thing I knew, they were in the hands of the police. I'm sorry. I didn't give him your name or address, but he does know the neighborhood you live in."

He hugged his pup like he would never again let him go. "Don't worry about it. Butkus, Ruby, Hershey, and I are leaving town tonight. Probably won't see you again." He interrupted his focus on Hershey and looked at me. "For what it's worth, I'm not a pusher, Doc. I supply a guy who sells the stuff to prisoners. He doesn't sell to kids." He sighed. "Sorry I got you into this mess. Can't thank you enough for everything you've done for us. I'll never forget you."

I nodded slowly and hoped that he would understand—the feeling was mutual. After a few last-minute instructions on Hershey's care, I said, "Take care of yourself, Luke." One last time, we shook hands. On his way out, he paid his bill—with cash.

Chapter 13

COWBOY JACK

It was a Tuesday night. Katy and I dried the boys after their bath. My pager rang. I called the number.

"Jim, it's Jack Archer. I've got a cow trying to deliver her calf. It's half in, half out. Looks like she's in trouble. My neighbor and I are trying to get her loaded right now. If I can get her to town, will you meet me at the clinic?" He sounded exhausted.

"Call me when you get to the edge of town. I'll be waiting for you," I said. I estimated that Jack and his neighbor, with a lot of luck, might get that cow loaded and be at my office in a little over an hour. I waited thirty minutes before I headed to the hospital.

Jack was a well-respected civil engineer and a friend. He was a quiet man in his mid-forties, tall and lanky with dark hair and a small mustache. He started with a small surveying company and turned it into a thriving business with three survey crews, a design staff of four engineers and five assistants, and a construction team of twelve workers. It was a curious thing that this successful man suddenly decided to try ranching as a hobby. Was he bored, needed more adventure in his life, or did he do it for his brother? Whatever the reason, Jack had no business raising cattle.

Jack's younger brother, an unemployed opportunistic slouch, convinced Jack that, with his cowboy knowledge and Jack's money, they would be rich ranchers. Jack bought some land and a hundred cows. He moved a trailer onto the site and hired his brother to watch over Jack's investment. It didn't take long before his brother decided that watching TV and drinking beer was a lot more fun than baby-sitting a bunch of stupid cows. By the time their first calving season arrived, Jack made the smart decision to cut his losses—he fired his brother.

It's critical that a rancher check on his cows twice a day during calving season in case of a birthing problem. With nobody living on the ranch and Jack's business demanding all his time, his cows were lucky if checked upon once a week.

I started my usual preparation for a cow with a difficult birthing. I filled a bucket with warm water and disinfectant and placed two O.B. chains and handles into the bucket. Each chain was three feet long, made of small chrome-plated stainless-steel links with a larger oval link at each end. The link on one end is passed through the link on the other end to form a loop which is slipped into the birth canal to snare one of the unborn calf's feet. With both chains firmly over the feet, fist-sized oval handles are attached to any link of the chains and used to pull the calf through a four-inch diameter tunnel.

From the large animal treatment room, through the open door, I could see the perimeter wall and electric gate that led into the yard

13 – Cowboy Jack

where we unloaded our large animal patients. The headlights of a truck announced Jack's arrival.

As the truck and trailer drove through the gate and into the yard, the unmistakable smell of death suddenly filled the air.

"Crap!" I said. I didn't have to examine the cow to know that her calf had been dead for some time and undoubtedly, the extraction of its rotten carcass was going to be an unpleasant challenge.

I closed the gate and watched this wannabe cowboy try, perhaps for the first time in his life, to back a trailer into an unloading area.

"That's good, Jack," I yelled, when after several unsuccessful attempts, the trailer finally contacted the gate of the receiving pen. Jack stepped out of his truck. He was a man very much out of his comfort zone. His shirt was soaked with sweat, his pants caked with mud. He wore a scarf over his nose and mouth.

"You don't look so good, Jack. You okay?"

"No, not really. I'm in over my head, Jim," he said and slowly shook his head. "I don't know when she went into labor. It may have been a while ago. She smells kinda rotten. I think the calf may be dead."

My first reaction was to say, "No shit, Jack!", but when I looked closer, I saw a guy who had already had a really lousy day. The last thing he needed was for me to rub salt in his wounds.

"Well, let's get her unloaded and we'll have a look," I said. I opened the trailer gate. A three-year old Hereford cow staggered out of the trailer and fell to her chest. Her beautiful brown eyes were sunken deep into their sockets and every breath she took was a labored effort. My first impression was that she was septic and dying.

"Let's take it easy with her, Jack. We don't want her going down in the alley on us," I said. After some gentle poking and prodding, the cow struggled to her feet and walked slowly down the alley and into the treatment room.

"Put that pipe behind her," I yelled as she entered the chute. I pulled on the handle that narrowed the sides of the metal enclosure and restricted the cow's movement. Jack slid a narrow bar through two fixed rings on both sides of the chute directly behind the cow's back legs to prevent her from backing up or kicking at me.

Two partially exposed feet stuck out of the back end of Jack's cow. I hoped they were front feet and that there was a head not far behind. Clostridial bacteria grow like wildfire in dead tissue and produce a sickening gas. I had delivered many dead calves in my career, but I had never faced one that smelled as bad as this one. I had learned to tolerate the bad ones, but this one was something altogether different, a heavy challenge on the nerve centers that connect the sense of smell with the vomiting center of the brain.

I slid plastic OB gloves over both hands and pulled them up to my shoulders. I stepped in behind the cow and reached blindly into a disgusting collection of rotting body parts. The exposed feet were indeed front feet, but there was no head in the birth canal. Without that head accompanying the front feet, there was no way she could deliver this calf.

13 – Cowboy Jack

Except for the front legs, I could feel no distinguishable body parts, only hair that peeled off the skin with ease and a chest tightly distended with gas that completely obstructed my entrance from the birth canal into the uterus.

"No way I can do a C-section on her, Jack. She won't survive it," I said as I struggled to suppress the urge to vomit. The green scarf that covered Jack's nose and mouth blended almost perfectly with the color of the rest of his face.

"You okay?" I asked.

"Uh…uh…Yup," he replied, desperate to keep his last meal from exploding into his scarf. Apparently, we shared the same urgency.

"Don't go too far. I may need your help. This calf is really decomposed. That could be to our advantage," I said. "It might just pull apart."

"Okay," he replied. He sounded like a guy who really needed to leave the room.

Mike and I kept a "calf puller" in our treatment room. It was a valuable device that we used as an aid when faced with a difficult delivery, but it was awkward and hard to operate single-handedly. Based on what I could see of Jack's face, I wasn't sure I could count on him for help, and I didn't want him fainting on me. I decided to proceed alone.

I looped a chain around one exposed foot and hooked a handle to it. My partner, Mike, had taught me a valuable trick. A skin incision completely around the leg just above the chain eliminated the toughest obstacle. The skin was much stronger than muscle attachments.

Dismemberment was now achievable by stretching the muscles to the point of separating them from bone. I was counting on significant tissue decomposition. It was like pulling a pillow out of its pillowcase. The key was not to get into an all-out, energy expending tug-of-war, but rather to apply consistent tension on the chain.

After several minutes of pulling, my head ached and my muscles burned like fire. I was just about to concede the battle when I felt something give. The skin just above my chain tore away from the underlying muscle. The muscles that attached the shoulder blade to the rib cage tore apart and the entire skinless front leg fell out onto the floor.

It was a good start. I looped my chain over the other exposed foot. I rested for a few minutes and began again. This one was not so easy. I pulled and pulled until I felt my muscles begin to fatigue. All muscles under the stress of continuous contraction eventually fatigue and lose their ability to contract. They simply run out of gas. It was the last thing I needed to deal with at this time. I took several deep breaths and pulled with what energy and strength I had left. Suddenly, the second leg tore free from the body and I landed on the concrete floor with the skinless leg on my chest. I laid there, nauseated, exhausted. My clothes were soaked, rich with the most indescribably awful smell I had ever experienced. What in the hell were you thinking when you decided on this for a profession, I wondered.

"That should give us a little more room to work with," I said. There was no answer.

13 – Cowboy Jack

"Jack?" Again, no answer. I looked over my shoulder. He was gone. I needed a break. I dropped the chain into the bucket and walked outside.

It was dark, but the moon was bright. Jack, on his hands and knees, leaned against the back tire of his truck. There was no sign of the green scarf. He retched, then heaved once, then twice, and again. It was a noble effort on his part. He had held on much longer than most would have, but in the end, they all lose it.

"Are you all right, Jack?"

"Just checking the air in my tires, Jim," he said as he cleared his throat and spit.

"Don't worry about it. Just sit there for a little bit. I got this," I said. I felt genuinely sympathetic.

I went back to the cow. She was weak. "Hang in there, girl. Don't go down. You do and I'll never be able to get you up." The muscles in my arms screamed. Time was critical. All my skills and experience, pulling, positioning, pulling again, making one small gain at a time, would all be for nothing if I ran out of strength and wasn't able to finish. I had to find that head in a hurry.

I shivered at the thought of going back in barehanded. All the showers in the world would not help. The smell would be with me for days and yet, I knew the plastic gloves would slow me down. From here on out, it was all about feel. Looks like I'm sleeping in the doghouse tonight, I thought.

I formed a loop with the chain, weaved it between my fingers, and plunged my entire arm into the birth canal. With the calf's front legs out of the way, there was much more room. My fingers found the curvature of the calf's neck. The head was turned back, the nose rested against the rib cage, a long way from my fingertips. Unless I turned the head to deliver nose first, this calf wasn't going anywhere. I reached and reached until I was up to my armpit in a foul mixture of liquids and solids powerful enough to make a maggot puke, but the calf's nose was too far away. Take a breath, I thought. Relax. Time for plan B.

I slipped the chain over and behind the neck and pulled it back to me from underneath. I threaded one end link through the other and pulled it tightly. The procedure was tricky, one-handed, but I had done it many times before. With a handle attached to the chain, I pulled on the neck with one hand while my other hand carried a second chain back in to find the nose. I pulled and reached, pulled and reached, each time, closer and closer until—there it was! I felt the tip of the nose. The muscles in my arms began to cramp. "Don't give up. You're almost there," I whispered. With my thumb, I peeled the loop off my fingers and over the calf's nose into the mouth. Get it past the teeth, I thought, or it'll come loose. Almost there, don't give up. The sharp teeth sliced into my fingers like razors as I forced the chain deep into the calf's mouth. There—you got it! With the chain looped securely through the calf's mouth, I slowly withdrew my hand, extended the loop behind both ears, and pulled the loose end of the chain tightly.

"Gotcha now!" I yelled as though I expected the cow to turn around and say, *Good job, Doc.* With that, I collapsed.

13 – Cowboy Jack

I sat with my elbows on my knees for several minutes, caught my breath, and willed my muscles to hang on. The smell no longer mattered. I was too tired to even notice it anymore. I gathered my feet under me. From out of nowhere came an extended hand.

"Let me help you up," Jack said.

"Good to see you, Jack," I replied as I rose to my feet. "We're almost home. One more pull and we've got it made. Are you with me?"

"Let's do this," he said. He took a deep breath and gritted his teeth. I hooked two handles six inches apart on the chain looped around the calf's head.

"You ready?" I asked. For the first time, I saw some fire in his eyes. He nodded.

"Nice and easy, Jack. We don't want to pull his head off. Here we go." We each grabbed a handle and started to pull. At first, I felt nothing. Then something began to give.

"Keep pulling," I exclaimed. The head slowly began to slip into position and then I could see the nose.

"This is it. Pull," I yelled. With every bit of strength that was left in us, we pulled. The nose was now fully exposed. Then came the rest of the head. Where she found the strength, I don't know, but at that very moment, the cow decided it was time to try or die. She pushed hard, and as Jack and I pulled with the last remnants of strength left in our bodies, the final remains of her once beautiful, now decayed, dismembered calf spilled out of her body, and splattered onto the ground.

The feeling is hard to describe, but it exists for any rancher or veterinarian who has ever experienced the difficult delivery of a calf. A live calf is obviously much better than a dead one, but dead or alive, when that calf finally squeezes out of that narrow tunnel and hits the ground, the sense of accomplishment, relief, and excitement are truly euphoric. I raised my fists into the air and laughed triumphantly. Jack managed to drag himself out of the room and heaved again.

I stood motionless for the next few minutes. Then I dragged the body parts out of the building and into the yard, grabbed a hose, and washed the rest of the stinky mess toward the floor drain. The air gradually became more tolerable. It was only then that Jack stumbled back into the room, walked directly to the sink, turned on the faucet, and splashed cold water on his face.

"You gonna make it, Jack?" I asked and chuckled.

"Yeah. I think so," he said and smiled. "What's next?"

"Well, first, we'll pump a few gallons of water into her rumen. She's dehydrated. Then we'll pump a couple of gallons of disinfectant solution into her uterus. That'll kill off the bacteria that are trying to kill her. With the calf out of the way, her uterus will begin to contract. Five ccs of oxytocin will get that started."

"You think she's going to make it?" Jack asked after we had finished treating her.

"Yeah, I think so. She's a tough old girl. The worst is over," I said. "Let's get her out of here before she falls."

The front gate of the chute opened and the cow staggered out into the alley and back towards Jack's trailer.

"Easy, girl," I whispered. "Almost there." When she reached the open end of the trailer, I held my breath. Ever so slowly, one foot at a time, she stepped into the trailer, and I closed the gate behind her.

Jack looked every bit as exhausted as his cow. He slowly pulled himself into the driver's seat of his truck and shut the door. Through the open window, he smiled. "Can't thank you enough, Jim."

"Don't thank me yet. Wait till you get my bill," I said and chuckled.

"Don't send the bill," he insisted. "I'll be by tomorrow to pay it. I'm going to take the day off. I need to spend some time with my real estate man." He turned the key and the truck's engine roared to life. He sighed.

"Don't know anybody who wants to buy a ranch, do you?"

MY FRIENDS WALK BAREFOOT

Chapter 14

FUNNY HOW THINGS TURN OUT

In the world of a veterinarian, it is often expected that at least one offspring will follow in the professional footsteps of their parent. I believed that prophecy—until now.

Roswell, New Mexico
1990

Friday nights were always family night at the Humphreys' house. The boys were allowed to stay up late and watch cartoons. John Thomas, JT as we called him, was five years old and very much into Bugs Bunny, Daffy Duck, and the Roadrunner. His collection of VHS tapes was enormous. His brother, Rob, three years younger, had little understanding of modern-day cartoon humor, but if big brother was in for a fun-filled night, he wasn't about to be left out.

As our family tradition dictated, we sat together at the table for supper before the start of the entertainment. There was nothing quite like a cartoon marathon as incentive for finishing supper in record time. JT hurried to help me clear the dishes as Katy wiped the food that didn't quite make it into Rob's mouth from his hands and face.

Then it happened. The only sound that could possibly disrupt our highly anticipated plans rang out loud and clear. I reached for my pager and saw a look of horror spread across JT's face. He understood perfectly what that sound meant.

"Oh, no!" he said and shook his head. Tears instantly filled his eyes. The message read: *Dog has large, barbed wire cut.* I called the number and made arrangements to meet my client and his injured dog at our hospital in 30 minutes. I hung up the phone and saw my son wrapped in his mother's arms. Tears streamed down his cheeks. I hated the never-ending disappointments that came with being on call, but it was part of the job.

"Why don't you guys get started. I'll join you as soon as I get back," I said.

"No, Papa. It's no fun without you," JT said as Katy held a Kleenex for him to blow his nose.

"This shouldn't take me very long. Maybe a couple of hours." I forced a smile.

"Hey, I have an idea. Why don't you go with Papa?" Katy said as she wiped JT's tears. "I'll bet he could use your help." She looked to me. Her eyes screamed for support.

"Great idea! What do you think, JT?" I asked.

He was quiet for a moment, then he smiled and nodded. "Yeah. I'll go with you, Papa."

14 – Funny How Things Turn Out

"Okay. Let's get going, Buddy. The sooner we get this done, the sooner we get back." JT hurried to his room and put on socks and shoes. I buckled him into his car seat and we were off on a grand adventure.

"Call me if you need help. Promise?" Katy yelled as we backed out of the driveway.

"Don't worry, sweetie. We'll be fine."

We arrived at the office ahead of my client and his dog. I stopped at the treatment room, gathered a surgery pack and some suture material. I heard a knock at the front door.

"Come on, son. Let's go see who's here," I said. A young man waited at the front door, his dog wrapped in a towel.

"Come on in," I said and opened the door. It was Jed, the oldest son of Brett Ellis, a long-time rancher client. He followed me back to the treatment room, set the dog down, and we reintroduced ourselves as Jed removed the towel. A jagged laceration extended down the dog's back from just behind her ears to the base of her tail.

Daisy was Jed's two-year old Dachshund. Her hair was too short to contain the blood that dripped from her back. It ran down both sides to her belly and to all four legs where it dried to a dark, shiny, sticky paste. Despite her gaping wound, Daisy wagged her tail and licked JT's hand as he reached to pet her on the head.

"Wow. That barbed wire saw you coming from a mile away, didn't it, Daisy," I said in an attempt to keep the conversation light.

Jed shook his head. "She can slip under most of our fences, but Dad and I strung an extra low strand around Mom's garden to try and keep the rabbits out. Hasn't worked very well. Daisy caught one of them chewing on a tomato plant and went after it. She tried squeezing under. Didn't quite make it."

I checked Daisy's vital signs. They were normal. "It looks nasty, but it's pretty clean," I told Jed. "Tomorrow, she'll look like Frankenstein, but when the stitches come out and the hair grows back, you'll never know it happened."

Jed held his dog while I drew a calculated dose of anesthetic and injected it into Daisy's hip muscle.

"Put her in here, Jed." I said. I opened a cage door. "It'll take a few minutes for her to fall asleep. Don't worry. She'll be fine. You can pick her up tomorrow morning."

"Thanks, Doc. Sorry I had to pull you out after hours," Jed said as we walked him to the front door.

"Not a problem, Jed. Say hi to your folks for me." We bid farewell to Jed, locked the front door, and walked back to check on Daisy.

"Come here, son," I said and lifted JT onto a counter next to the prep table. "This will give you a front row seat." I retrieved my anesthetized patient from her cage and carefully placed her on the steel grate that covered the tub of our surgical prep table. Tonight, it would serve as the site where I would suture the wound. I extended her tongue out of her mouth so that I could continuously evaluate its color. Then I washed the dried blood from her body.

"JT, I need you to keep an eye on the color of Daisy's tongue. Make sure it stays bright pink. Let me know if it changes at all, okay?"

"Okay," he said with a confident head nod. Then he appeared to be confused.

"What other colors can it be, Papa?" he asked.

I had to think about that one for a minute. "Well—don't worry about it, son. Anything other than pink is bad."

JT took his responsibility seriously. His curiosity urged him to move closer, to make sure he had a clear view of the pink tongue. That also gave him a much clearer view of the blood as it slowly liquefied and dripped off Daisy's unconscious body into the stainless-steel tub below the grate and disappeared down the drain.

The sound of the electric clippers sparked JT's curiosity. He leaned forward. As the clippers removed the hair, the bruised, edematous fibers of exposed muscle glared under bloodless, jagged edges of skin.

"Are you okay, son?" I asked as I peeked over the top of my glasses.

"Uh, I think so," JT said with a slightly hesitant voice. He paused for a moment.

"Yeah, I'm okay," he said with decided confidence.

With the wound clipped and surgically prepped, I opened the instrument pack, donned a pair of sterile latex gloves, and covered Daisy with a sterile drape that exposed only the laceration and of course, the bright pink tongue. I had to make sure my little partner could do his job properly.

I stood next to the grate, over my patient and prepared to cut away the torn, dead edges of skin with a pair of surgical scissors as my brave son watched. With careful precision, I removed a two-millimeter strip of ragged skin along the edge of the laceration and left behind a pristine edge of healthy tissue, filled with life, confirmed by the blood that began to flow again.

"How we doin', JT?" I asked as I placed the first suture. There was no answer. I placed a second suture.

"Son?" Still no answer. I looked up. JT's eyes were fixed on the pile of blood-soaked gauze sponges at one edge of the drape. His sun-soaked, beautiful tan face had turned a light shade of green.

He began to lean. I dropped the instruments on the drape and with complete disregard, I reached with every inch of my arms and back. I caught my son just before his head struck the unyielding floor.

I laid him face up on the floor, placed a dry towel under his head and a moist one on his forehead. He began to regain consciousness. My bloody gloves had inadvertently painted JT's face, neck, hair, and his t-shirt.

"You okay, Buddy?" Despite his lingering delirium, he nodded. "Close your eyes and relax. We're going home soon." I changed my gloves and finished suturing a fifteen-inch laceration in a time worthy of a new Guinness World Record.

It was dark when we arrived home. Katy and Rob waited for us on the front porch. I helped JT out of the truck. As the dim porch light slowly revealed his hair and face, Katy's smile turned to a look of horror. "What the . . .?" she exclaimed.

"It's okay. It's not his blood," I said instantly, attempting to defuse the situation. "We had a little mishap."

14 – Funny How Things Turn Out

"Didn't we, Buddy? Come on, let's get you cleaned up," I said. "How about cartoons tomorrow night?"

The following day, we decided to give our cartoon evening another try. I had learned early in my career, not to plan family activities when I was on call. Nevertheless, we were confident that tonight would be different. We popped the popcorn and dimmed the lights as JT set up the VHS. No sooner had we sat down to watch Bugs Bunny and Yosemite Sam duke it out when my pager rang. Once again, I called the number.

"Jim? I'm so sorry to call you on the weekend." Ruth Simpson was perhaps the sweetest lady I had ever had the privilege of calling my client and my friend. She had been a widow for ten years. A mother of five and a grandmother of twelve, she lived alone on the family farm on the edge of town.

"It's Rosebud, Jim. She's been in labor for over three hours. I think she's got one stuck." Rosebud was one of Ruth's favorite Duroc sows. An experienced pig farmer, Ruth watched her "kids" very closely, but I had never known her to panic. If Ruth said Rosebud was in trouble, I wasn't about to argue.

"Be there in fifteen minutes, Ruth." I walked back into the TV room and sighed. "Well, guess what?"

JT looked at me through sad eyes. "You want me to go with you, Papa?"

"No, son. You guys watch Bugs so you can tell me all about it later, okay?"

"How about you, Rob. You wanna go with Papa?" Katy asked.

He broke into his ear-to-ear Rob smile and threw his hands in the air. "Me, Papa!"

"What do you think?" Katy asked, with a look of concern. I suspected she hadn't expected Rob to agree and had second thoughts about letting him go after the last bloody incident.

"Why not. He'll be fine. Ruth will be thrilled with the company," I said.

"Come on, little bug. Let's go."

Ruth Simpson didn't operate a typical pig farm. There were no crates, no pens full of mud and flies and amazingly, the offensive odor was minimal. "I don't know why we humans should think we're the only animals in the world who need social interaction," she had once said to me. Her sows all shared the same spacious, clean barn with access to an outdoor fenced yard for basking in the sun. As birthing time approached, Ruth guided the expectant mother to a corner of the barn where a bed of fresh straw had been curtained off by short walls constructed of hay bales.

Ruth's property was surrounded by a tall fence, interrupted by a single entrance with a cattle guard to keep any animals from wandering too far. True to her hospitable nature, Ruth left the outdoor lights on and the barn doors wide open so that I could see where to go. The evening was warm. I took Rob's shirt off and left him wearing only his diaper. I scooped him out of his car seat and we walked into the well-lit barn.

Ruth stood next to Rosebud, her denim shirt and coveralls soaked in sweat. "Jim! Thanks for comin'. Who is this gorgeous boy?"

"This is Rob." Children usually seek the security of a parent when in the presence of a total stranger, but not Rob. He gave Ruth that Rob smile and extended his arms as if to say, "Take me."

"Hi, little Rob," she said as I handed my son, in his diaper, into her arms. "I got everything ready for you, Jim. She's over here."

I peeked into Ruth's labor and delivery corner where Rosebud lay on her side, panting. Next to her was a bucket of water, a bar of soap, a bottle of disinfectant solution, and a tube of lubricant gel. I washed the pig's perineum with soap and water. I scrubbed my hands and arms, sprayed them with disinfectant, and knelt behind Rosebud. Ruth sat on a hay bale. My son bounced on her knee to the rhythm of J.J. Cale's "Call me the Breeze," on the radio.

With a handful of lubricant, I laid on my side and slowly inserted my hand into Rosebud's birth canal. I was close to reaching the full extent of my arm when I felt two small front feet. The baby's head was folded back. The nose rested on its right shoulder, a common scenario in birthing problems. If feet and head are not in the birth canal together, even the strongest of uterine contractions cannot expel the baby.

In the background, I heard Ruth. "Hey, little Rob. You gonna be a pig doctor like your daddy some day?"

With extended fingers, I reached between the front legs, located the baby's shoulders, and gently pushed the body back into the uterus. The exercise was contrary to Rosebud's contractions. She pushed hard and forced the little pig against my hand.

"Easy, girl," I said. I held my ground until she stopped pushing, then continued to repel the fetus. Finally able to reach across the head, I hooked my forefinger behind the baby's nose and flipped the head back into position. "Gotcha," I whispered triumphantly as Rosebud gave a hard push that shot my arm and baby number one out of the birth canal. I scooted back on my elbows until I was on my knees and picked up the baby pig which immediately began to squeal.

"Here you go, Ruth," I yelled over my shoulder.

"Uh oh. I gotta go to work, little Rob." Ruth sat Rob on the bed of straw against a hay bale, an arm's length away from the action, took the baby pig from me, and dried it aggressively with a towel. By the time I focused my attention back on Rosebud, she had pushed again, and two more babies lay on the ground. The piglets instantly jumped up, shook violently, and squealed. Rosebud pushed again and again, and in a matter of minutes, six newborn pigs scurried about. They shook themselves dry and screamed at ear-piercing decibels.

Rosebud was exhausted, decided to take a break, and relaxed.

It suddenly occurred to me to check on Rob. My two-year old boy sat where Ruth had placed him wearing a diaper and nothing else. Bodily fluids of every known color and consistency covered his legs, chest, and face. A string of placenta hung from a lock of his blonde hair. Two of the baby pigs had determined that Rob was their mother and instinctively fought to be first to nurse from his toes.

"You okay, little bug?" I asked.

Rob had a unique facial expression that told the world he wasn't happy. He lowered his chin, furrowed his eyebrows, and pushed his lower lip out as far as it would go. In a very deliberate voice, he said, "Don yike it!"

I searched for a dry towel. There were none. I grabbed the cleanest one I could find and wiped his face. That did nothing more than smear spots of blood into patterns that resembled war paint. The noise and confusion combined with Ruth's laughter each time a new baby hit the ground were all just a bit more than this little boy could take. I lifted him off the ground and hugged him tightly as tears streamed down his face. "Let's go home, little bug."

"Pretty sure she's not done, Ruth. She'll need to rest for a while. Do you still have that oxytocin I gave you a while back?" I asked.

"Sure do," she replied.

"Give her half an hour to rest, then give her five ccs in the muscle," I instructed. "That should kick her uterus back into gear. Don't think she'll have any more problems. Call me if you need to."

"Get after it, kids," Ruth said as she positioned each baby pig next to one of Rosebud's teats. Then she stood and gave me a hug.

"Thanks, Jim."

She kissed my son on his forehead. "Little Rob, you come see me again real soon, okay?"

Katy and JT waited on the front porch as we approached the driveway. "I was beginning to worry about you," Katy said.

I gathered Rob in one arm and walked toward the front door. Our son's bloody face and body slowly slid into the light. Katy saw him and put her hands on her hips.

"Seriously!"

"He's fine. I promise. Let's don't forget whose idea this was, okay," I said in an effort to salvage the night.

She looked at me without saying a word, scooped Rob from my arms and said, "Did you have fun, baby boy?"

Rob gave his mother a hug. Then came that classic look. "Don yike it!"

I smiled sheepishly. "I'll tell you all about it later. Come on, bug. Let's hit the shower and get you to bed."

Las Cruces, New Mexico
2007

The three-hour drive over the mountains from Roswell to Las Cruces for a concert had become a common and much-anticipated activity for Katy and me in the latest chapter of our lives. The boys were both in college at New Mexico State University. JT, a junior and Rob, a freshman, were both in the university band and had asked us to meet them at their favorite restaurant before their much-anticipated jazz band concert.

"What time do you have to be at the music hall?" I asked.

"We have plenty of time. Concert isn't 'til eight," JT said as he looked at his watch. "You and Mama should probably be there half an hour early. It's gonna be packed. Dr. Romero wants all the horns there at seven. We have a few wrinkles to iron out. We're playing one of your favorites, Papa—'Birdland'. Guess what? I have a solo."

"Wow, JT!" I said. "That's awesome. Can't wait, son."

14 – Funny How Things Turn Out

"I probably better go back with JT," Rob said as he finished the last bite of his steak. "I need to help the sound guy get my drums miked. He's a really nice guy. Just doesn't know what he's doing. I get to try out my new Ride Cymbal," he said with excitement.

He looked at his big brother and puffed up his chest. "I have a solo, too."

Katy gazed at her boys, her elbows on the table, her chin cradled in the palms of her hands. Her face beamed with pride.

"Wow. Look at you guys. After all those AP math classes I made you take and Papa dragging you around on calls, I was so sure one of you would be an engineer," then glancing at me, "and the other, a veterinarian. Instead, here we are. Both of you on your way to becoming professional musicians."

I set my knife and fork down, and smiled. "Yeah, funny how things turn out."

Chapter 15

DANCER

It was quarter past five on Friday afternoon and fifteen minutes left on the clock before our office closed. It had been a long and stressful week and I looked forward to a relaxing weekend. The phone rang.

"Dr. Humphreys," Roseann said. Our receptionist had that look on her face that told me it was bad news. "I'm sorry. I have Ms. Stewart on line one. She has a colicky horse. She asked for you."

Crap! I thought. I don't believe this. I was so close to getting out of here. Why couldn't she have waited for just a few more minutes?

"Lee? It's Jim. What's goin' on?" I asked in the most pleasant voice I could muster.

"Jim!" Her voice was on the edge of panic. "It's Dancer. She's got a bad case of colic. I can't keep her up. I need you as soon as you can get here."

"Try to keep her walking. I'm on my way."

Lee Stewart had been a client for years. She was middle-aged, tall, and muscular with short blonde hair. As far as I knew, she had never married, had no family to speak of, and few friends. She had one passion in life—Hunter/Jumper competition. Lee was a champion rider. Together, she and Dancer competed across the country and had won so many times that Lee had long ago lost track of the number of ribbons and trophies.

Dancer was a twenty-five-year-old chestnut thoroughbred mare that Lee had raised from a four-month-old filly. She had beautiful brown eyes, a long flowing mane, and a tail that reached almost to the ground. Dancer was Lee's only child.

I hung up the phone and shook my head. It was my partner Mike's weekend to handle emergency calls. Just fifteen minutes and Dancer's problem would have been his to answer. I knew Mike would step up and take the case if I asked him to, but Lee had asked for me. Like it or not, this call was my responsibility.

It was nearly six when I arrived at Lee's place. Her twenty-acre property was completely fenced. The east half was a dirt field with a challenging obstacle course designed to keep both Lee and Dancer well trained and in good shape. On the west ten acres was a modest house with a nice lawn and tall trees, a six-stall stable, and an adjacent hay barn. The sign at the entrance read, *Stewart Stables—Riding classes—Boarding.* I drove through the main entrance and saw Lee as she struggled to keep her mare walking.

Colic is nothing more than a bellyache, but in a horse, it's extremely dangerous. It usually starts when food travels through the intestines without sufficient liquid to keep it moving. There are several areas in a horse's intestinal tract where a ten-inch diameter bowel funnels down to a three-inch diameter quickly. If dry food reaches one of those areas, it can easily block the flow. Gas builds up behind the

15 – Dancer

impaction and causes distention of the bowel and excruciating pain. Because horses are intolerant of pain, most with colic will drop to the ground and begin to roll. A horse rolling on the ground with loops of bowel distended with gas is an impending prequel to a bowel *torsion*, that is, a loop of bowel that flips over on its own axis and cuts off its blood supply. Without surgery, the horse with a bowel torsion will die.

I stepped out of my truck and saw Dancer as I had never seen her before. The mare sweated profusely and stomped her front feet on the ground as she tried desperately to deal with her pain. I hurried to the mobile pharmacy in the back of my truck, drew heavy doses of painkiller and tranquilizer into separate syringes, and administered them intravenously to the mare. Within minutes, Dancer began to relax. Her labored breathing eased and her relentless obsession to lie down and roll subsided.

I lifted her upper lip and exposed her gums. They were dark purple in color, not healthy pink like they should have been—a bad sign. I pulled a stethoscope from my breast pocket and listened to her heart rate. Despite the painkiller, it was over one hundred beats per minute, three times normal—another bad sign. Finally, I listened to her abdomen and hoped to hear any sound of gas rumbling through the bowels which indicated that things were still moving. There was none. Not even a squeak. Dancer was in serious trouble.

"She's bad, isn't she, Jim?"

"Yeah. She really is, Lee. If getting her to a surgeon is an option, we need to go now." Colic surgery on a horse is something not every veterinarian is capable of doing. Our closest equine surgeon was four hours away.

"Do you think she'll survive the trip?" she asked.

"I don't know. She could go down in the trailer and then she'll really be in a mess. First thing I'll have to do is see if I can get hold of anyone who's willing to take her. It's Friday afternoon, you know. It'll be expensive, Lee. Very expensive."

Lee kicked at the dirt and shook her head, frustrated by her dilemma. "What should I do," she cried out. She paced and paced and slowly came to grips with the hard facts. "I love her to death, Jim, but she's twenty-five years old and I don't have that kind of money. Surgery is not an option."

"Understood. Looks like it's just you and me," I said as I struggled to maintain a reassuring smile. "We'll have to sweat it out as best we can."

I went to my truck and gathered a five-liter bag of intravenous fluids, a drip line, and a large bore catheter. Lee and Dancer stood next to a post that carried the electric cable to Lee's house. I found a nail set high in the post and hung the bag of fluids on it. I placed the catheter into Dancer's jugular vein, connected the fluids and drip line, and ran the fluids into her blood stream as fast as they would go. I passed a tube through Dancer's nose into her stomach and pumped a gallon of mineral oil through the tube. With any luck, the oil might help break up the presumptive bowel impaction.

"Do you think she has a chance?" Lee asked.

"Of course she does."

15 – Dancer

"What kind of chance?"

I sighed. "Not very good."

Tearfully, Lee nodded—a confirmation that she knew we were in for a rough night.

"Lee, I'm going home to get something to eat. I'll be back in an hour. Try to keep her up," I insisted. I jumped into my truck and sped home.

"Papa," JT yelled as I walked through the front door.

Rob danced around in circles. "Papa's home. Papa's home."

"We picked out a movie just for you," JT said. "It's your favorite. *Daffy Duck's Fantastic Island.*"

I couldn't help but laugh. I knelt, gathered them both tightly in my arms, looked at Katy, and shook my head. "Don't have much time," I whispered. "Got a bad colic."

She took a deep breath, released it slowly and frowned. "But you're not on call."

"I know," I said and shrugged my shoulders. "It just happened."

Katy nodded and forced a smile. "Okay, boys. Bath time. Papa needs to eat."

I ate quickly, then helped Katy dry the boys off after their bath as tears streamed down their cheeks.

"Why do you have to go, Papa?" JT whimpered.

"Well, there's this beautiful horse, JT. Her name is Dancer." I patted his belly. "She has a really bad tummy ache and I'm the only one who can fix her. We'll watch the movie tomorrow. I promise. Okay?"

With his lower lip pushed out as far as it would go, he nodded. I kissed them both. "I'll see you tomorrow, boys."

On the way back to Lee's house, I called Kenny Winkler. He had a backhoe and was one of the few people around willing to make a house call to bury a dead horse.

"Don't think she's gonna make it, Kenny. Wanted to alert you just in case," I said. "If she dies, I'm sure Lee will want to bury her behind the barn."

"Don't worry about it, Doc," Kenny replied. "You can call me anytime. I know where Lee lives. I can be there in an hour. Sure hope she makes it. Lee does love that mare."

For the next four hours, I flooded Dancer's veins with tranquilizer and painkiller as it became more and more apparent that perhaps I had lost the battle. As quickly as one bag of IV fluids emptied, I attached another bag to continue the flow.

"How much of that painkiller can she have?" Lee asked.

"As much as it takes."

It was just after midnight when Dancer suddenly, and for no apparent reason, stopped hurting. Her pain was gone, turned off as quickly as a light switch. She held her head up, her ears forward, and her breathing relaxed. The sweat that had rolled off her body like a fountain suddenly dried up.

Lee noticed the change immediately. "What just happened, Jim? Her pain is gone. Why?" she asked, her voice balancing sorrow and excitement.

I wasn't sure what the answer was. I examined the mare closely and after careful consideration, finally answered, "Well, it could be an intestinal impaction has just broken loose."

"That's a good thing, right," Lee said. Her voice was suddenly full of hope.

"Yes, Lee. That's a very good thing."

"So, why aren't you excited?"

I was still unsure about what had just happened, but I gave careful thought to my next answer. "Well . . . there's another possibility. She may have just perforated a bowel."

Lee looked at me, confused. I wasn't sure how to proceed, but I wasn't going to hide the truth. I took a deep breath and let it go.

"A bowel perforation releases all the gas that has been distending the intestine into her abdomen. The pain is gone instantly." I paused. "The problem is . . . a bowel perforation will also release the rest of the intestinal contents into the abdomen. It's like a ruptured appendix, Lee . . . only much worse.

"What then?" she asked anxiously.

"Bacteria will spread like wildfire. The ensuing infection creates massive inflammation in the abdomen. It's called *peritonitis*. The pain will be back in a hurry, and with a vengeance. Bacterial toxins will invade her blood stream. We call that *septicemia*." I paused, searching for something positive, an encouraging word to throw into the conversation. There was none. I bowed my head. "She'll die."

Lee buried her face in the palms of her hands and shook her head. "I don't know what to do."

I didn't know what to do either. Should I hug her? What could I do to make this any easier? Unfortunately, not much. "Right now, there's nothing to do," I said. "She's not in pain. We need to tie her to this post and let the fluids run, let the mineral oil move downstream, and hope for the best. I'm going to give her some more painkiller and I'm going home. Bring a sleeping bag out here if you need to, but lie down and get some rest," I insisted. I ran to my truck, grabbed a piece of paper and a pen, and began writing as I walked back toward Lee. I handed her the paper.

"Here's my home phone number. The next few hours will tell us a lot. I'll wait for your call," I said.

As I drove away, I knew the night was young, that I would be back soon, and that Dancer would probably never see the light of day. It was one o'clock in the morning when I crept into the house. Katy and the boys were curled up in our bed fast asleep. Gently, I carried my sons back to their beds, tucked them both in, crawled in next to my wife, and turned out the light. Three hours later, the phone rang. It was Lee.

"Give me some good news, Lee," I said as I struggled to shake off the cobwebs.

"She was okay for a while," she said. "I managed to sleep. She woke me up when she fell to the ground. She pulled her IV catheter out. There's blood everywhere. I can't get her up. I think it's time to call it quits, Jim." She sounded completely spent.

"On my way," I said.

15 – Dancer

There was a heavy mist in the air as I drove past the gate toward the barn. The moon was shrouded in clouds and there was but one dim light mounted on the post next to the mare. Dancer lay flat on her side, breathing heavily. Lee knelt next to her and gently wiped the mare's face with a moist cloth.

I walked over to the mare and knelt next to Lee. She looked at me, eyes tired, her cheeks stained by tears and dust. "Is there anything you can do for her?"

I carefully lifted Dancer's upper lip. Her gums were gray and dry. Her belly was distended with gas and her skin was wet and cold. I looked into her eyes and sensed that she was trying to tell me something. Something like, *I've had enough.*

"I'm so sorry, Lee. There's only one way we can help her now . . . It's time."

Lee was silent for a long time. She wiped the tears from her eyes.

"Then I owe it to her. I don't want to see her in pain anymore. Would you please put her to sleep?"

I knelt, silent for a moment, then stood and walked to my truck. I opened the door to my mobile pharmacy, pulled open the top drawer, and reached far back for the bottle of euthanasia solution. I hated the stuff. It was fluorescent pink and thick like motor oil. Every time I had to do this, I realized what a luxury it was for veterinarians, unlike physicians, to be allowed to end a patient's suffering with a simple injection. Yet, each time I reached for that bottle of *pink juice*, I felt profoundly defeated.

I grabbed a sixty-milliliter syringe and a fourteen-gauge, three-inch needle. I filled the syringe with the lethal solution and walked back to Dancer and Lee.

"Maybe you'd better go inside and let me handle this, Lee."

"No. We've been in lots of tough spots together over the years. She never abandoned me. I'm not leaving her now," she said with conviction.

I nodded, stepped up to Dancer's shoulder and knelt next to her. I glanced at Lee. I saw a person, completely exhausted, both physically and mentally. The muscles of her face sagged and her eyes were blank, devoid of any expression.

I sighed. "Here we go."

I detached the needle from the syringe and removed the protective plastic cap from the needle. I pressed my right thumb against the mare's neck directly over the jugular vein. The pressure partially occluded the flow of blood, which dilated the vessel and made it more visible in the dim light. With my left hand I gave the needle a firm, quick stick through the skin and into the lumen of the distended vein. Blood instantly squirted back through the needle confirming that it was properly placed. I removed my thumb from Dancer's neck, which allowed blood to flow freely down the pulsating track. I attached the syringe to the needle and delivered the unforgiving solution into the mare's bloodstream. I tossed the needle and syringe aside and whispered, "Go to sleep, girl."

The euthanasia solution raced down Dancer's jugular directly into her heart. Lee hung her head and wept. It took approximately five seconds from the time the last milliliter of pink poison started down its deadly path until the mare lost consciousness. There was no struggle, no violent convulsion—only the sound of freedom as Dancer took a deep breath, exhaled, and died.

It was eight in the morning when I arrived home. Katy had made waffles. She and the boys sat at the breakfast table when I walked in. J.T. turned to face me.

"Papa! Did you fix Dancer?"

"I did, son. She's not hurting anymore."

MY FRIENDS WALK BAREFOOT

Chapter 16

OSTRICH HEAVEN

Ben Garner was a big man who would never be caught without his cowboy hat, western shirt, blue jeans, and boots. His wide belt was cinched tightly to help support his bad back, the result of years of hard labor and hauling a substantial beer belly. Every breath he took was an effort which always ended with a pronounced wheeze—the price of smoking two packs a day.

I sat at my desk looking through patient records when I heard someone enter the front door. I immediately recognized that loud and unmistakable voice.

"Has Dr. Jim come in yet? I need to see him right away."

We had good receptionists over the years, but none quite as good as Roseann. Her voice was strong and confident. "Hi, Mr. Garner. Dr. Humphreys is in the middle of finishing the morning procedures just now. Would you like to have a seat, or do you need to run an errand and come back in an hour or so?"

Actually, she hadn't seen me come in and had no idea what I was doing.

"I'll wait. I really need to see him," he said emphatically.

Roseann quietly slipped out of the reception area and into my office. "Good morning. Ben Garner is up front. He's insistent about seeing you right away. He's sitting on the bench with his hands in his lap and his legs crossed like he's about to pee in his pants."

"Does he have an emergency?" I asked.

"I don't think so," Roseann said as she looked over her shoulder. "I think he's just really excited about something, or maybe he's upset. Hard to say. You know Mr. Garner."

I walked into the reception room and Ben jumped out of his seat. "Jimbo! How the hell are you?"

He hadn't changed a bit since I had last seen him.

"Hello, Ben. How've you been, man?" I shook his trembling hand.

"Jimmy boy, I gotta new project and I need your help. What do you know about ratites?" His face was full of anticipation, like a kid who had just asked his mother if he could sleep over at a friend's house.

"What's a ratite?" I asked, after a long pause. I knew what a ratite was, but I let that sink in for a bit and then I smiled. "Just kidding, Ben. What's going on?"

He took a deep breath, regained his composure, and spoke slowly. "Jim, I'm in the ostrich business."

Somehow, I wasn't surprised. Ben had tried his luck at several careers over the years—ranching, selling real estate, building houses, and touring with a local band. Each time, he dove in knowing little if anything about what he was doing, but always with amazing confidence and enthusiasm. Rumor had it that he had made and lost several fortunes.

"You're kidding me, right?" I said with a sly smile.

"I'm serious, Doc. I've done my research. These birds are gonna make me a rich man, and I want you to be my vet."

"Great," I said as I struggled to hold a smile. I didn't know a thing about ostriches, but I wasn't about to let him know that.

"Here you go." He handed me a book—*Ratites, A to Z.*

"Tell me what you've got," I said as I looked at the front cover.

His eyes filled with excitement. "I got a great deal from a rancher in Texas. This guy's been breeding ostriches for four years now. I spent a week with him learning all the ins and outs of the trade. I bought four breeding pairs for $50,000 a pair, ten yearlings for $2,500 apiece, thirty-month-old chicks for $1,000 apiece, and he threw in some fertilized eggs for free."

I didn't know what to say. I really admired Ben's courage, but historically that courage had not fared well. He had just bought a quarter of a million dollars' worth of birds that as far as I knew, were valued for only two things—leather boots and feather dusters. Those were going to be some very expensive boots.

The temptation to say, "Are you nuts?" was overwhelming, but that wouldn't be very professional. "Wow. Sounds like a heck of a deal. So, what's the plan?"

"I'm building pens right now. The birds arrive next week," he said. "I've got a consultant coming in two weeks to help me get things up and running. In the meantime, we need to do our homework. Read that book and I'll call you when the birds get here. You can come out, look around, and tell me what you think."

"I'll tell you what I think. You're a brave man, Ben. Call when you're ready for me. I'm always up for a new adventure."

He skipped out of the office. Roseann looked at me with a broad smile.

"Sounds like fun, doesn't it."

"Ask me later. I have some serious studying to do," I replied as I stared at my new book.

The following Monday, Ben called. "The first bunch got here about an hour ago, Jimbo. The rest are due later today. When can you come out?"

"How about tomorrow morning? Say, nine o'clock," I said.

"Sounds great," he said. "Don't worry about bringing anything special. We're not givin' no shots or nothin'. I just need you to look things over."

I was used to venturing into uncharted territories not knowing where they may lead. I had diagnosed and treated snakes, lizards, bears, and mountain lions, but this time, as I drove into Ben's driveway, my nerves acted up like never before. I had read the book and learned a little about ostrich husbandry, but knew nothing about their anatomy, physiology, or pathology.

Ben had built a beautiful home on the edge of town, surrounded by pecan trees and a gorgeous, well-manicured lawn. Behind the house was a five-acre tract which had once been an alfalfa field. That land was now compacted dirt surrounded by an eight-foot high, four-rail

16 – Ostrich Heaven

pipe fence with small-gauge web wire that was buried in the ground and extended to the top rail of pipe. Ben had divided the lot into ten equal-sized pens, each with its own water supply, feed trough, and covered shelter to provide shade and protection from inclement weather.

I walked toward the main gate and passed a crew of five men hoisting Ben's new sign onto two metal posts. The big letters, professionally carved out of the solid oak background and painted bright white, read: OSTRICH HEAVEN.

Ben waved. "Over here, Jim." We met and shook hands. He escorted me into a small metal building that was centered at the entrance to the pens. A radio played "Nine to Five." Dolly Parton sang loud enough to be heard from anywhere in the yard.

"The radio is on twenty-four seven. Apparently, ostriches are just like me. They love music," he said. "It relaxes them."

I wasn't a fan of the genre myself. "Are you sure they like country?" I asked. "Maybe you ought to try some rock and roll."

"Naw, I don't think so," he said with a chuckle. "Come see my new incubator."

It looked like a giant bread maker, a low temperature oven with a large glass bubble for a lid.

"I spared no expense on this little beauty. It turns the eggs automatically at whatever time interval you set, real important. Temperature and humidity are controlled," he explained. "It even has a gadget that candles the egg to let you know if it's fertile and how the embryo is doing. Pretty slick, huh?"

"Wow. Pretty cool, but I don't get it. Why don't you just let the birds hatch the eggs?" I suddenly felt like I ought to have known the answer to that question.

"Are you kidding?" he exclaimed with a frown. "Haven't been studying much, have you? Can't afford to take a chance on an egg getting stepped on and crushed. A fertilized egg is worth a thousand bucks. Problem is that the rooster guards the eggs. He'll kill anything that gets close to them. The hen will lay her eggs in a nest on the ground. As soon as that egg is in the nest, I gotta get it outta there."

"How do you intend to do that?" I asked.

"Haven't figured that part out, yet. The guy that's bringing my fertilized eggs next week is gonna teach me all sorts of crap I have no idea about. Come on. I'll show you the place."

We walked into a pen of young chicks. Like a tourist guide, Ben explained one of the inherent problems with raising ostriches. "These crazy birds will eat anything that's shiny. They love metal and glass. I've got to make sure the place is clean all the time. If I'm out in the yard, I'll be drinking my beer out of a paper cup. They get hold of metal or glass, it's *adios amigos*. Just hope the neighbors don't throw any trash over the fence."

"Speaking of neighbors, what do they think about an ostrich farm sitting in their back yard?" I asked.

"I don't know. I guess I'll find out soon enough. I sold every one of them their land, so I suppose they shouldn't have a whole lot of reason to bitch."

16 – Ostrich Heaven

I thought about that statement for a good while. I couldn't find the logic in it, but decided to keep my mouth shut.

We were instantly surrounded by dozens of little fuzz-balls that pecked at our boots and darted back and forth between our feet.

"Kinda cute, aren't they," Ben said. "They've got plenty of water and their feed trough is always full, but every time I step into this pen, they're all over me. I guess they think I'm their mama." I looked across the yard at one of the adult hens.

"Yeah, I think you're right, Ben. I can see the resemblance."

We stepped into a pen of yearling birds. The older birds were closer to our height and weight. They had begun to grow the classic, beautiful, brown feathers. Their necks and legs had stretched like bamboo shoots. Their eyelids were paper-thin and stretched with each blink to cover huge brown eyes. These teenagers gave us a much different reception than their younger siblings.

"These guys are a lot more suspicious. They're real curious, too. Stand still for a minute," he whispered.

The adolescent chicks walked toward us, one very careful step at a time until they were just out of reach. They stood motionless until one of us moved and sent them scurrying at full speed in the opposite direction. They were intrigued by Ben's silver watchband. One of the chick's curiosity overpowered his good sense and the bird reached out, pecked at the watch, then ran away.

Ben laughed. "See what I mean? That's why I don't wear my wedding ring out here. One of these rascals is liable to take it right off my finger."

We entered a narrow alley adjacent to the breeding pairs. The females were smaller than the males and not nearly as colorful. The male birds had much darker feathers and brighter red skin on their legs and neck. The first two pens each had one pair of adults—a male and a female. The third pen had two females with one male, and the last pen, a single male.

I was curious about the distribution in the last two pens. "How come this guy is by himself?"

"He's the main reason you're here, Jimbo. None of these birds are insured yet. If one of these females were to kick at him and break one of his legs, I'd lose a ton of money. He's my pride and joy," he said as he puffed up his chest. "Just look at him. He's a good six inches taller and nearly a hundred pounds heavier than these other males. I call him Big Bird."

I looked at him closely. He was gorgeous and huge, close to eight feet tall and weighed well over 300 pounds. His feathers were black as night and the skin on his neck and legs shone like a bad sunburn.

"I didn't know you were a Sesame Street fan, Ben."

He cocked his head. "A what kinda fan?" He stopped and thought about it for a bit before he made the connection. "You mean the kids' show? Oh, I get what you're saying. You mean Big Bird? Know what? That never occurred to me. Tell me the truth, Jimbo. Have you ever in your life, seen a bigger bird?"

"No Ben. Never. I get it," I replied as I stared at the giant avian.

"I've got a form I need to fill out to get him insured. There's a part for you to fill out, too," he said with a smile. Uh oh, I thought. Here it comes. "They want to know a few simple things," he continued, "like . . . oh, you know . . . that his heart and lungs sound good, skin is healthy, good eyes. Simple stuff like that."

"Right," I said as I felt myself being sucked in. "So, is he friendly?"

"Friendly? Oh, hell, no. He's feisty," he replied. "See that claw on his front toe? He has the strength in his legs to shoot that claw right through your skull or split your rib cage wide open. The good news is he's not guarding any eggs right now. We'll be all right."

"You got any body armor?" I asked with a chuckle which was meant to sound like I was joking, but I truly wasn't.

"No," he replied. "I got some safety helmets ordered, but they ain't here yet. We'll be all right. These guys can only kick forward. If we stay behind him, we'll be all right."

I looked at him, quite certain we were not on the same page. "This is just getting better and better. I don't suppose he's just going to stand there while we sneak up on him from behind, is he?"

"No, not exactly. I need you to distract him while I sneak up on him." He pulled a sock from his back pocket. "I'll reach over his back from behind, grab him by the neck, and pull his head down to the ground. He can't kick with his head on the ground. Then I'll pull this sock over his head and turn him loose. When he can't see anything, he'll settle right down. Piece of cake, Jimbo."

I stood tall, struggled to remain calm, and tried to reinforce that I was not one bit intimidated by what he was asking me to do—I wasn't very convincing. "Are you sure about this, Ben? Have you seen this done before?"

"We'll be all right." He smiled.

I took that as a *no*. I walked to the fence and grabbed it with both hands.

Big Bird started to cluck, extended his wings, stamped his feet, and charged the fence. I jumped backward, fell on my butt, then sat there and trembled as I tried to catch my breath.

"That's his aggressive mode," Ben roared.

"No shit!" I yelled, professionalism set aside given my present state of mind.

Ben helped me to my feet, walked over to the only tree in the yard, and broke off a branch. He turned and walked toward me as he swung his hips and sang with the radio, "Don't tell my heart. My achy, breaky heart." He peeled off all the leaves except for those at the tip and handed me the branch. "Are you ready?"

The branch was a bit shorter than my arm. I took it from him. "What's this for?"

"That's just in case he charges. Wave it in his face and it'll keep him off you," he smirked.

That was the last straw. "Pretty sure of that, are you? Are you nuts? I'm not going in that pen with this maniac!" I held the stick at arms-length. "This stick is supposed to protect me? It's half the length of his leg, Ben!"

"I'll be right there with you, Jimbo. Don't worry." He smiled. "We'll be all right."

All right, my ass, I thought. I took a minute to consider my options. I entertained the idea of taking off my boots, thinking I might have a better chance scaling the fence barefoot, but decided that might be a stupid idea after all. If I was going to die, it might as well be like a real cowboy.

Big Bird's pen was square, fifty feet long and wide. Ben opened the gate and we stepped inside. The ostrich paced back and forth along the opposite fence. In the middle of the pen was his feed trough, a heavy metal structure, two feet wide and ten feet long, attached to a stand about four feet off the ground.

"Keep that trough between him and us," Ben whispered.

"Right," I replied. We walked, ever so slowly toward the middle of the pen. Big Bird's impatience grew. My heart beat faster and faster. I felt sweat run down my back, as always seemed to be the case on my harrowing adventures.

"Let's split up," Ben said. "I'll go left, you go right. Try to draw him toward you. Whatever you do, keep him on the other side of that feed trough."

"I know, Ben, I know." I reached the right edge of the trough at the exact time that Big Bird decided he had had enough. From across the pen, he charged straight at me. I had no idea what to do. I shook the branch in his direction as a hard as I could. He got close enough to jump into my back pocket in what seemed like a fraction of a second. Suddenly, he came to a dead stop. He was just out of my reach. I was well within his. His eyes, big as golf balls, stared at me, curiously, as if he wondered, *What in the hell do you think you're doing with that silly stick, little man?*

I caught a glimpse of Ben as he circled around the trough and closed in on Big Bird from behind. I was amazed at how quickly and quietly the big man moved. He reached the ostrich before the bird had a chance to respond. With his left hand covered by the inverted sock, his right hand reached over Big Bird's back. He threw his weight forward until he was able to grasp the bird's long neck. Startled, the ostrich swung his head around, stamped his feet, and hissed at his attacker. Ben's right hand shot its way up the long neck and reached the head. Big Bird's reaction was too late. With his left hand, Ben grabbed Big Bird's beak and his right hand pulled the sock over the ostrich's head. He released his grip and jumped back.

My heart pounded. I expected the worst. Nothing happened. The ostrich shook his head violently for a few seconds to free himself of the sock that blinded him. Then he stood tall and silent.

"Ha! I told you so," Ben yelled triumphantly.

I couldn't believe my eyes. Big Bird's head darted back and forth as he looked for the light, but he didn't fight or panic. He just stood there.

"He's all yours, Jimbo," Ben said as he stepped back and presented his trophy to me.

I took a minute to gather the little bit of courage I had left, walked toward the scariest bird I had ever seen in my life, and gently rested my hands on his back and breast. He was a magnificent animal. His feathers were soft and billowy. I moved slowly as not to startle him.

Gently, I started at his head, still covered by the sock and worked my way down his neck, across his back and down his breast and legs, and felt for any abnormal lumps or bumps. His skin was rough and stretched tightly over massive, well-defined leg muscles. I quietly pulled my stethoscope from my breast pocket and placed it under his wing. I wasn't sure where best to listen for a heartbeat, but I could feel the brachial artery under the heavy wing, against the back of my hand as it pulsated slowly, powerfully, and rhythmically. I checked his feathers. They appeared healthy. I searched for anything that might represent a problem and found nothing.

"Seems to be in great shape," I said. "I need to look at his eyes."

"Here, let me have him," Ben whispered and grabbed the bird by the head. "Ready?"

Before I had a chance to think about it, Ben pulled Big Bird's head to the ground and gently removed the sock. I knelt next to him, once again eye to eye with this beautiful but scary creature. He blinked once, twice. His eyes were huge, the lids, almost transparent with healthy, tortuous blood vessels that streaked both laterally and vertically. The lashes were long and dark like they had been painted with mascara. I moved his head from side to side. His pupils responded well to the light and his corneas were clear with no visible abnormalities.

"I think we're done," I said. I started to plan my escape route when Ben suddenly and without warning, turned the ostrich loose. It was too late to run. On my hands and knees, I looked up and saw two giant bird feet, each with an incredibly ominous toenail pointed straight at me. He had us dead to rights, and for a brief second, I wondered what it would feel like to be impaled.

Big Bird stood tall and looked down at us as if to say, *are you quite done?* Then he turned and slowly walked away. Ben and I looked at each other and without a word, we agreed it was time for us to leave.

"Well?" Ben asked as we walked out of Big Bird's pen.

"Just like you said, Ben. 'Piece of cake.'"

"I told you we'd be all right." He laughed and slapped me on the back. "Jimbo, we're gonna have a helluva lot of fun."

Chapter 17

BRENDA'S SONG

Brenda had worked for us for the past two years and was about to start her senior year in high school. She was tall and slender with long brown hair, hazel eyes, and a sweet smile. Brenda was a natural athlete—the star of both the volleyball and basketball teams, and one of the best high school students we had ever hired. She was quiet, but confident, hard-working, and afraid of nothing. I attributed her courage to a tough, early childhood. Her parents were killed in a car accident when she was six years old. Brenda's grandparents gave her a new home on a small farm on the west edge of town, filled with love, discipline, and purpose. She thrived.

"He's a Great Pearlenese, Doc. Best damn sheepdog in the world. I paid $5,000 for him. I can see most of my pastures from the upper deck of my house. Got one pasture that borders a big arroyo. The coyotes love it. Lots of places to hide out. I lost twenty lambs in that pasture last year to those varmints. This dog's gonna change that."

Carl Davis was a third-generation sheep rancher—and a real grouch. He was a short man, maybe five-five with a scraggly beard, long tangled grey hair, and a potbelly. His shirt was never tucked in and his boots desperately needed new soles. He owned a ranch about twenty-five miles directly west of town. His wife had divorced him. His two sons and a daughter, all grown and gone from the ranch, had not the slightest interest in ranching. "They didn't want to grow up to be like their ol' man," Clay Summers once told me. Clay was Mr. Davis' ranch foreman.

I had to think about it for a minute. I hadn't seen the dog, but I suspected what my client had bought was a Great Pyrenees, a guard dog that was originally bred in the high mountains between France and Spain to protect sheep from the wolves.

I looked into the back of Mr. Davis' stock trailer and saw a young dog lying on a bed of straw. He was perhaps just shy of a year of age and growing fast. I estimated he already weighed over a hundred pounds. He was snowy white except for the edges of his eyelids, his nose, and lips, which were black as coal. His hair was long, thick, and straight. He had a huge head and beautiful eyes, brown and sad.

"I'm gonna leave him with you for a week, Doc. I have to take a load of ewes to Dallas. I'll pick him up on the way home. I need you to check him over, give him any shots he needs. He's not mean, won't give you no trouble. He leads pretty good on a leash, but here's the deal, Doc. I don't want anybody lovin' on this dog. No pettin' or huggin'. If you socialize this dog, you'll ruin him. Just feed and water him and leave him alone."

I had several clients who owned a Great Pyrenees. They were all gentle giants, great family dogs, but not worth what Mr. Davis had paid for this one.

"I didn't realize these dogs were so expensive, Mr. Davis."

17 – Brenda's Song

"That's 'cuz you're used to seeing silver dollars. I bought me a gold coin. These damn US breeders have ruined these dogs," he said with contempt in his voice. "Turned them into pets. Something for their kids to crawl all over, hug, and kiss. I had this dog shipped from Barcelona, Spain. He's guaranteed to kill any coyote, wolf, or mountain lion that gets anywhere close to his flock."

I glanced over my shoulder. Brenda stood behind me and peeked into the trailer. "Brenda, you think you can find a run for Mr. Davis' dog?" I asked.

"No!" Mr. Davis yelled. "He needs to stay out here in a horse stall. He gets no special treatment. Is that understood," he snarled at Brenda.

Brenda looked at him with a smile and without so much as a hint of being intimidated. She stepped into the trailer, put a leash around the dog's neck, and led him to a clean horse stall.

"He's all yours, Doc," Mr. Davis said as he shuffled back to his truck. He heaved himself into the driver's seat and slammed the door shut.

"I don't like that man," Brenda whispered, as Mr. Davis drove away. "That stall is really hard dirt, Dr. Humphreys. Can I put a blanket in there with him?"

"Well, we're not supposed to." She looked at me with pitifully sad eyes. "Okay, Brenda. Put a blanket in there with him."

The rest of the week was different than most. It was Brenda's last week of summer vacation. She worked full time and our paths typically crossed at least a dozen times a day, but not this week.

Each time I asked a staff member, "Where's Brenda?" the answer always seemed to be the same.

"Uh, not sure. I think she's out back." I didn't want to check up on her for fear I might find her huddled up in a corner of the horse stall with Mr. Davis' dog.

On Friday afternoon, once again, I asked our receptionist, Roseann, "Have you seen Brenda?"

"I think she took Placido for a walk," she replied.

"Placido? Who's Placido?" I suddenly realized that, maybe, I didn't want to know the answer to my question.

Roseann realized she had unintentionally disclosed a deep, dark secret. Her face turned bright red. "Uh, that's what Brenda named Mr. Davis' dog," she answered.

"She's did what? She named Mr. Davis' dog? Placido?" I asked in disbelief.

"Yeah, Dr. Humphreys. You know, Placido. Like Placido Domingo. He's a Spanish tenor."

"I know who Placido Domingo is, Roseann," I said with a hint of impatience.

"Brenda thought the name fit him well," she said and gave a soft sigh. "After all, they're both Spaniards, they both have gorgeous eyes, and it just so happens that Placido Domingo is Brenda's grandmother's favorite singer."

"Oh yeah? Well, something tells me that Mr. Davis is not a music lover," I said with disgust.

"Placido is," she said with a sheepish smile.

17 – Brenda's Song

"What do you mean?"

"Brenda sings a lullaby to him every evening before she leaves. Don't tell her I told you," she whispered.

I took a deep breath, closed my eyes, and imagined what Mr. Davis might think of our irresponsible care of his killer dog. "Oh, my goodness. If that dog goes home and decides that letting his coyote buddies serenade him is a lot more fun than chasing them off, Mr. Davis will have our hides."

"Chris!" I yelled down the hallway. "Go find Brenda and tell her to put that dog back in his stall . . . now!" I went to my office and closed the door in frustration.

It was Brenda's turn to feed and clean that weekend and my weekend to do morning and afternoon treatments. I could always count on her to be there to help me with treatments as well as make sure every animal was fed, had plenty of water, that the clinic was spotless, and didn't smell.

Sunday morning, I drove to the office earlier than usual to study the schedule for the next week. I sat at the reception desk when I saw Brenda drive into the parking lot. She got out of her pickup and peeked through the glass of the entrance door. She immediately realized that I had arrived ahead of her. She hadn't expected me to be at the office that early and a look of horror spread across her face as I stood and met her at the door.

"Okay. "Where is he?" I asked.

She walked slowly to the passenger side of the pickup and opened the door. Placido stepped out.

It took all I had to keep my cool. "Brenda! Really?"

"I'm so sorry, Dr. Humphreys. I knew he was going to the ranch tomorrow. I figured if he was destined to live in an open field, exposed to cold, rain, and snow with no one to talk to except a bunch of stupid sheep, he deserved one night in a comfortable home."

I could see tears welling in her eyes.

"We sat on the front porch for hours while I played my guitar and sang to him. I wrote a song for him," she said proudly. "He really loves it. He kept bumping me with his nose to play it over and over again." She sighed deeply. "He slept at the foot of my bed."

Whether it was intentional or not, she did a first-rate job of melting my heart. "What did your grandparents have to say?" I asked.

"They love him. I told them it was just one night, but I didn't tell them the whole story. Please don't fire me."

Fire her? We had had lots of kids work for us over the years. Most of them were good, but then, there was Brenda. She was that once-in-a-lifetime kid who knew and did her job well. She never complained, and somehow, made everybody's day a little brighter.

"Nobody's going to fire you, Brenda." I chuckled. "Even if I wanted to, I can't afford to fire you. I expect you to come back here and buy this practice someday." I sighed. "Have you completely forgotten what Mr. Davis demanded of us?"

"No, sir. He said I was to leave him alone."

"Exactly. Somehow, I don't think he would consider sleeping at the foot of your bed . . . acceptable."

17 – Brenda's Song

She allowed herself a devilish grin. "I won't tell anyone if you don't."

It seemed like anything she said drew a smile from me. "Fair enough. Put him up and don't you dare take him out again until Mr. Davis gets back."

"Yes sir."

The following day marked the start of the new school year. Brenda rushed back to the clinic after her last class. She wanted to be there to say goodbye. I watched as she led Placido into Mr. Davis' stock trailer. It took every bit of her strength not to kneel next to him and hug him. She struggled desperately to hold back tears. Then she walked quickly out of the trailer and straight into the clinic. I knew her heart was broken, but I also knew that in time, she would be all right. Soon there would be student council meetings, volleyball practice, and homework to keep her mind busy.

Time passed and so did the seasons. Fall became winter and winter turned into spring. Mid-April found me in the farm and ranch store buying some dripline for a new group of trees I had planted when I heard a familiar voice.

"Hey, Doc." I turned and there was Clay Summers, Carl Davis' ranch foreman.

"Hello, Clay," I said as I reached to shake his hand. "How the heck are you, man?"

"Been busy, Doc. We just barely finished fixing fence line when the ewes started lambing. How have you been?"

"Doing well, Clay," I replied. "Speaking of lambing, how has Placi . . . uh, Mr. Davis' new dog been working out?"

Clay smiled. "You know what, Doc? In all the years I've worked for that old man, he's made lots of bad decisions, but buying that dog was not one of them. That's the greatest guard dog I've ever seen," Clay boasted. "He hadn't been in the field for two weeks before a coyote got a bit too close. Poor beast was either awfully bold or awfully stupid. That dog ran him down and killed him on the spot."

"You're kidding me," I said.

"That's only half the story, Doc. There's a big, tall berm in the middle of that pasture. It used to be part of a dam that was built to catch the monsoon rains." He laughed. "Back in the day when it used to rain. That dog dragged that coyote to the top of that berm for the whole world to see. The blood trail was over a hundred feet long. It was almost like he was making a statement," Clay continued. "Letting everybody know that there was a new sheriff in town, and they best not mess with his sheep. Damnedest thing I ever saw. We haven't lost a single lamb this season. Hey, I better go, Doc. Good to see you."

"Good to see you too, Clay. Give my best to Mr. Davis."

I considered telling Brenda about my conversation with Clay, but decided that old wound didn't need to be reopened.

Three weeks later, we heard the tragic news on the radio. Local rancher, Carl Davis had been killed in a freak accident on his ranch. Details were sketchy.

17 – Brenda's Song

Two weeks after we received that news, Roseann stepped into my office. "Clay Summers is up front. He came to town to pay some ranch bills. Sounds like he's moving. He wants to say goodbye."

"Ask him to come on back, Roseann." In the blink of an eye, a tired, sad ranch foreman stood at the door to my office.

"Come on in and have a seat, Clay," I said. He sat down and took a slow deep breath, as if it were the first time in a long time that he had been allowed to relax.

"I can't stay long, Doc. Just wanted to thank you for everything you've done for us." We sat for 30 minutes while he gave me all the details of the accident and about the plans for the ranch. "I've got a job offer up north I'm gonna look at," he said.

"I wish you all the best, Clay. Keep in touch," I said. We shook hands and he walked away.

At the end of the day, the entire staff, all dying of curiosity, gathered in my office, and I relayed Clay's story. Mr. Davis had been checking his pastures on his 4-wheeler ATV. He caught a steep hill at a bad angle. The machine rolled over on top of him and killed him instantly.

None of his children wanted anything to do with the ranch, and so, the bank was in the process of putting it up for sale. Carl's neighbor had decided to buy all the sheep. Clay and his men had spent the last week gathering and shipping.

I looked at Brenda. "The last pasture they gathered was Placido's. Apparently, he stood guard the entire time to make sure nobody was left behind. When he was satisfied that all his flock were penned, he disappeared."

"What do you mean, he disappeared?" Brenda asked.

"Well, according to Mr. Summers, as they were loading the sheep onto trucks, one of his guys noticed Placido walking across the pasture. Clay assumed he wasn't going anywhere so he didn't give it a second thought. That was two days ago. He hasn't been back since. Clay put the word out to the neighbors. Nobody's seen him."

"How the hell can you not see a giant-sized, snow-white dog walking across open land!" Roseann yelled with exasperation.

"Why would he do that?" Brenda asked.

"I don't know," I said. "Maybe he just figured his job was done."

I was finishing some medical records when Brenda came into my office. She had been crying.

"Dr. Humphreys?"

"Come in and sit down, Brenda."

"What's he going to do, Dr. Humphreys? Where's he going to go? Who's going to take care of him?" Her voice trembled.

"I suspect he's going to be just fine, Brenda," I said with confidence. "He's a tough dog. He reminds me a lot of someone else I know. Don't you worry. He'll find a new family. Just like you did." I paused for a bit and handed her a Kleenex to blow her nose.

"Tell you what, Brenda. The last time he was seen, he was headed due East. Maybe you should leave the porch light on tonight. You never know. After all, he does love your song, doesn't he?"

Chapter 18
Rani (*raw knee*)

"Dr. Humphreys, do you have a minute?" Roseann asked.

"Yeah. What's up?" I asked as I looked up from the lab report I was reading.

"There are a couple of gentlemen who would like to speak with you. You gotta see these guys, sir," she said with a strange smirk.

Two men stood in the waiting room. The one to my left was thin, about six feet tall with straight black hair, an olive complexion, and brown eyes. He wore a maroon silk shirt and tight black pants. To his left was a big man, a very big man, perhaps six feet, six inches tall. His bushy eyebrows hung on a heavy skull. His head was shaved and blended into his shoulders by way of a thick, muscular neck. His arms were the diameter of my thighs and his enormous shoulders and chest stretched his bright orange shirt to its limits.

"Good morning, gentlemen," I said and extended my hand. "I'm Jim Humphreys."

"Doctor, my name is Marco. I am pleased to meet you," said the smaller man as he shook my hand. He pointed to the big man. "This is my little brother, Bruno."

Bruno took a step forward, clicked his heals, and bowed. "Is my supreme pleasure, Dr. Humpher, Humpheree?" he asked with a thick, Eastern European accent.

"My name is Jim, Bruno. Just Jim," I said and smiled. I reached to shake his hand and felt mine swallowed by his. To my surprise, and relief, his handshake was firm, but not too firm.

"What can I do for you?" I asked.

Bruno gave way to his brother who began their story. "My brother and I own a circus. It is small. We travel all over the country. Perhaps you have seen an advertisement announcing our arrival in your city?"

"As a matter of fact, I just saw a poster in the grocery store last night. Barcini Brothers Circus. Is that you?" I asked.

"Ah, it seems the man we pay to advertise is doing his job well, yes?" He sighed. "Doctor, we are a small troupe. Our artists are skilled, entertaining. Our show is very good." Slowly and deliberately, he ran his fingers through his dark hair. "Unfortunately, the star of our show is not well. She has not been able to perform for several weeks. If she cannot perform, reviews of our show are not as good as we need for them to be. Word travels fast. Audiences get smaller," he said.

I understood what he was getting at. An artistic company of their size was most likely operating on a shoestring. They needed full audiences to survive. "Mr. Barcini . . ."

"Please, call me Marco," he insisted, with a closed fist over his heart.

I smiled and with a shallow bow, I said, "Marco, I don't understand. Why have you come to see me?"

18 – Rani

He looked at his brother, then at me. "Doctor, we have a Bengal tiger."

I was stunned. No circus, large or small, that I had ever seen, had a Bengal tiger. They were too dangerous. "You have a . . . you have a Bengal tiger?"

"Yes. We bought her three years ago from a man who . . ."

"He was a monster!" Bruno shouted in anger.

Marco gently placed an open hand on his brother's shoulder to calm his rage. "When we bought her, she was unable to support any weight on her left front foot. These bones," he pointed to the long bones of his hand, "were broken. I knew this man. Bruno is correct. He was a monster. People said he beat his animals with a baseball bat when he was displeased. I suspect he sold her so cheaply just to get rid of her. We could not splint or even bandage the foot. She was wild."

Bruno stepped forward. "It took one year, Dr. Jim, for I earn her trust. Another year for she allow me to touch her foot. The bones healed, but not good. She has bad days and not so bad days. After show, I . . . how you say?" he asked, as he looked at his brother.

Marco said, "Bruno wraps her foot in an ice pack after every show. She has done very well until this month. Perhaps the weather."

"She lets you do this?" I looked at both with astonishment.

"Only Bruno. He is careful, moves slowly, speaks softly. Bruno and Rani have developed a very special bond, Doctor. He knows her well, and she trusts him," Marco said. "She knows he will not allow her to perform if she is in pain."

Tears welled in Bruno's eyes. "Please, Dr. Jim, will you come?"

My partner, Mike, was on a country call, treating a horse. I looked at Roseann, who in turn, looked at the schedule.

"You're free, Dr. Humphreys. I'll reschedule your morning appointments," she said. "Christine and I'll cover for you." It was a comfort to know I had a receptionist and a technician of such calibers as Roseann and Christine. They made my job so much easier.

"Okay, gentlemen, let's go," I said. "I assume you're setting up at the fairgrounds?"

"Follow me, please," Marco said with a burst of excitement.

I drove into the fairgrounds and saw people running in every direction, some carrying equipment, others pulling on ropes. In the middle of an open field, a huge tent began to take shape. At the far end of the field was a line of trucks and trailers. Marco led me around and behind the massed vehicles where I first saw the arena. It looked small, but became more impressive as I drove up to it.

I walked to the massive enclosure. Panels constructed of one-inch diameter steel bars were secured together forming a circular arena. One panel had been adapted to attach to a smaller cage, five feet wide, six feet high, and ten feet long.

Lying quietly in the middle of her ring of steel was the most beautiful animal I had ever seen. Bright orange stripes rippled across her body with strokes of black down her sides and patches of white on her face and underbelly. She must have been at least twelve feet long from the tip of her nose to the tip of her tail, I thought. I estimated her weight at about 350 pounds. She had a massive head with large brown eyes.

18 – Rani

Marco stood at attention as if announcing the President to Congress. "Doctor, let me introduce you to Rani."

I stared at her for a long time. Her beautiful colors, muscular body, powerful jaw, and majestic presence were mesmerizing. "Rani? That sounds East Indian."

"You are correct, Dr. Jim," Bruno said. "It means *Queen*."

I was so captivated by her beauty that I was unable to take my eyes off her. "Very appropriate, Bruno," I said.

Rani became acutely aware of my presence as I slowly walked the perimeter of her arena. Her cautious eyes were fixed on me. "Bruno, do you think she would let me examine the foot?" I asked.

"No, Dr. Jim. This, she will not do. Do you have something for to make her sleepy?"

"I do, but it has to be injected into a muscle. I have to get closer than this."

"Is not a problem," Bruno said. He pointed to the smaller cage. "She is used to cage. She is there for travel and when we set up arena for show."

"Okay. You get her into her cage and I'll get what I need to anesthetize her," I whispered, as not to further arouse any suspicion in Rani.

From the mobile pharmacy of my truck, I grabbed the pole syringe—a thirty-nine-inch fiberglass stick with a rubber grip at one end and a twelve-milliliter syringe at the opposite end. I attached a sixteen-gauge needle to the syringe and drew up a calculated dose of anesthetic agent.

Rani was now in the smaller cage, her head moving slowly to the left, then to the right as her eyes meticulously assessed every detail of her new surroundings.

"Bruno, I need you to distract her," I whispered. With his soft, reassuring voice, Bruno was able to coax her to one end of the cage. I crept quietly behind Rani. I struggled to control a trembling hand and carefully passed the jab stick through the bars of the cage until the needle was within several inches of the tigress' hip muscles. I drew a deep breath and released it slowly. With the force of my back and shoulder behind the jab stick, I thrust the needle deep into Rani's back leg.

Despite her confined space, she threw her head and neck over her shoulder and lunged at me with a deafening roar that made every hair on my body stand on end. I checked the syringe. It was empty. The anesthetic had been delivered as planned.

"We have about ten minutes before she'll be asleep. We need to get her back to my hospital for x-rays," I said. "I assume we have flat-bed truck to load the cage onto?" It was a critical detail I had failed to address before I had started down this "never before travelled road."

Marco and Bruno looked at each other, then back at me. "There is no flat-bed, Doctor," Marco said. "When we travel, Rani and her cage are in there," he said and pointed to a sixty-foot tractor-trailer.

I looked at the eighteen-wheeler and shook my head. "Well, that won't work. Any alternative?"

"Yes! I get cargo van," Bruno yelled as he ran off in the opposite direction.

18 – *Rani*

Cargo van? The cage won't fit, I thought.

After I felt confident that Rani was unconscious, I took a few seconds to run my hand across the fur on her chest as if to confirm that it was real. It wasn't soft like cotton, but rather satiny, each hair shaft shining like colored glass between my fingers.

Then, in an act that I was quite certain was completely against all local, state, and federal safety regulations, four men, all grunting and groaning, loaded a 350-pound, man-eating Bengal tiger from her cage into the back of a standard cargo van and headed up Main Street toward my hospital.

I called Roseann. "Have Christine fire up the x-ray machine and processor. We'll need the gas anesthetic machine, too."

Mike and Santiago had just returned from their country call and were unloading equipment from Mike's truck when we drove through the gate that led to the back entrance of the hospital. I jumped out of my truck and called to them for help as Bruno backed the van up to the door.

Mike opened the back doors to the van and stood back. "What the hell?"

"I'll explain later, Mike." The five of us carried Rani out of the van and into the building, to the x-ray room. Christine waited with the anesthetic machine and the largest endo-tracheal tube we had. She took one look at the size of Rani's head, said, "I don't think so," and ran to retrieve a face mask.

I ran my fingers between the metacarpal bones of Rani's bad foot. The foot was huge, the nails, long and sharp. I could feel scar tissue between the bones. We took several x-rays from different angles. The pictures were dramatic. The second and fifth metacarpals, the most medial and lateral bones of the foot, had healed and remodeled with little complication. The fractures of the third and fourth metacarpals, the central bones of the foot, had been severely displaced and had healed with large bone spurs that I suspected put pressure on the nerves and tendons. Activity undoubtedly created more inflammation and pain.

Mike and I studied and discussed the x-rays for a long time. It was a nasty looking foot.

"What can you do?" Bruno asked.

"Well, I could refer you to a specialist, an orthopedic surgeon," I replied. "There's a lot of scar tissue. That makes surgery difficult. It'll cost a lot of money."

"Can you do anything to make for her more comfort?" Bruno asked.

I sensed his anxiety and I wished that I could honestly give him good news. I looked back at the x-rays and shook my head. "Maybe, but I'm not sure for how long."

"You are a good man, Dr. Jim. Please, whatever you can do." He looked at me with trust and confidence.

"How's she doing, Christine?" I asked.

She listened intensely with her stethoscope. "She's doing fine," Christine replied.

I reached into a drawer and grabbed twelve-ml and three-ml syringes. I attached needles to each one and drew up separate drugs.

"What are these?" Bruno asked.

"This is dexamethasone. It's a very potent corticosteroid—short acting," I said, as I held up the large syringe. "This other one is another cortisone, Depo-Medrol, for long-acting effect . . . hopefully four to six weeks."

While Christine prepared the foot, I reviewed the x-rays and then I strategically injected both solutions into several areas of the foot where I thought they might produce maximum benefit.

"That's it," I said. "Let's get her home."

"Uh, Dr. Humphreys?" Christine said with a hint of concern. "About getting her home?"

I looked at her and wondered what the problem was. Christine didn't miss anything, but the expression on her face told me that I had. It took a minute and then it hit me.

Isoflurane had revolutionized the use of gas anesthesia. It was ultra-safe. Its most redeeming qualities were the speed with which a patient could be induced into an unconscious state and more importantly—the rapid recovery phase. The injectable anesthetic I had given Rani at the fairgrounds had surely worn off. As soon as that mask came off her face, she would be waking up—in a hurry.

I evaluated my options. I considered giving Rani another dose of injectable anesthesia, but the additive effect of multiple doses of injectable anesthetics can be tricky and dangerous. I decided it was best to get her home as fast as possible.

"Is there a problem, Doctor?" Marco asked.

I struggled to disguise my embarrassment. "Uh, we're going to have to take the back roads to the fairgrounds. The distance is a bit longer, but there are fewer stop lights, less traffic, fewer people." I hoped that I sounded confident.

"I don't understand," Marco said.

"Well, you see, it's going to take us about fifteen minutes to get Rani back to her cage. Our anesthetic machine is not portable." I struggled with my next statement. "We won't have much time after we pull this mask off her face before she wakes up."

"How much time?" Marco asked with a hint of concern in his voice.

I wiped the sweat from my upper lip. "Oh, probably . . . uh . . . maybe ten to fifteen minutes."

"Oh! I see the problem," Marco said.

I could tell he felt a sense of alarm, but he did well to disguise it.

"Okay, here's the plan," I said. "Santiago, I'm gonna need my truck out front. Bruno, you back the cargo van as close as you can get to the front door. It'll be faster and easier to take her out that way. Once we have her loaded, I'll take the lead. There are three traffic lights. If I have to, I'll try to stop cross traffic and let you through. Mike, do you think we can get the large gurney down the hallway?"

"Yeah, it'll just fit. I'll get it," he said. With the plan well understood, everyone jumped to their respective assignments.

Suddenly, Roseann appeared at the door that led to the hallway. I recognized the look on her face—more problems.

"Guess who just walked in," she said. "Mrs. McDonald . . . and Rebel."

"You're kidding me!" I exclaimed.

"Oh, how I wish I was," she said, "and no, she did not have an appointment. She wants you to check a little mole on top of Rebel's head. I told her it was going to be a while. She doesn't mind waiting," Roseann said calmly.

Rebel was Mrs. McDonald's Jack Russell Terrier, a ten-pound mass of muscle who could not hold still or be quiet for longer than a few seconds at a time. He had a high-pitched bark that typically went on and on from the minute he stepped into our office until he was out the door. He was a sweet dog who loved everybody and everything, except for—cats! Rebel hated cats so much that he simply couldn't be in the same room with one without lunging at it. Although Mrs. McDonald seldom had an appointment, when she and Rebel entered the building, if the waiting room was full, they were always escorted to the first available exam room.

"This has gotten a bit complicated, Roseann. I gotta go back to the fairgrounds," I said. "Oh yeah, and we need to go out the front door."

"Really?" Her eyes widened. She glanced down the hallway. "I guess I better get Rebel into an exam room."

"Naw, leave him alone. We'll zip past him before he knows what's going on," I said. "When we're out the door, ask Mrs. McDonald if Mike can look at Rebel's mole."

Mike had returned with the gurney followed by Santiago and Bruno. I checked to make sure everybody was in position.

"Are we ready?" I asked. Christine removed the mask from Rani's face. The gurney was only twelve inches off the ground and ran on hard rubber wheels. Slowly, we lowered Rani onto it. It was just long enough for her body.

"Somebody keep her tail from dragging," I said. "Let's go."

We entered the hallway. I could hear Rebel. *Bark, bark-bark, bark-bark.* The wheels of the gurney rumbled down the hallway. Although he couldn't see us, Rebel became increasingly aware of something headed in his direction. The cadence of his bark increased. *Bark-bark-bark, bark-bark-bark.* We rounded the corner into the waiting room. Rebel lunged forward and jerked on the end of his leash. *Bark-bark-bark* and then, in a single bound, he flew back into Mrs. McDonald's lap. His pupils were dilated and his body shook like a leaf battered by the wind. For the first time in his life, Rebel McDonald was at a complete loss for barks. I could only imagine what he was thinking. *Wow! That is one big kitty!*

Bruno ran ahead and had the van ready when we rolled out the front door. Together, we lifted Rani into the van. Bruno jumped in and sat beside her.

"What are you doing, Bruno?" I asked.

"I go with her."

"Bruno, I don't think that's such a good idea." He looked at me with a kind but determined expression.

"Dr. Jim. Will be okay. We go now."

The cab and cargo area of the van were separated. There would be no way for Marco to talk to Bruno. We slammed the doors shut.

"Follow me, Marco, and stay as close as you can." He nodded and we were off. I felt the beads of sweat collecting on my forehead. I had seen the violence with which a horse often wakes in the dark from an anesthetic-induced sleep. I didn't want to imagine what a 350-pound Bengal tiger might do. It was a mistake to let Bruno ride with her. I picked up speed as we approached the first traffic light.

"Please stay green, please, please stay green," I prayed. It did. One down, I thought. Two more to go. I looked in the mirror to check on Marco, who was giving new meaning to the word, "tailgating". Had he been any closer, we would have locked bumpers. Traffic was light and for the first time that I could recall, I hit all three green lights.

I checked my watch as we flew past the front entrance to the fairgrounds. Twelve minutes. Maybe she would still be groggy. Marco rolled his window down and yelled something to a couple of his crew. They ran to Rani's cage and pulled open the sliding gate as Marco backed up as close as he could get, allowing space to open the van doors. I jumped out of my truck and ran to the van.

"I'll get one door, Marco, you get the other," I whispered.

He looked at me and took a deep breath. "Be careful, Doctor." My heart pounded as if it might burst through my chest as I reached for the door. We looked at each other, signaled with a nod, and opened the doors. Bruno sat and faced the open doors, his legs crossed. Rani lay next to him on her chest, her head held high, her eyes wide open. She purred as Bruno ran his fingers through her hair and massaged her neck.

Casually, Bruno stepped out of the van and gestured toward the open cage. "Come on sweetheart. Let's get you some breakfast."

Chapter 19

Rani Part II

The Magic of Life

It was a short fifteen-minute drive, but I had never felt more nervous. I had allowed a man, a client, to ride in an enclosed van with a Bengal tiger who was rapidly recovering from anesthesia. Rani and Bruno had a special relationship, but I had no idea how the tigress would respond if she awoke to the smell of live flesh.

Marco and I were profoundly relieved to see Bruno alive and smiling. Rani rose and slowly stepped out of the van and into her cage—on three legs. I glanced at Bruno who shook his head and looked away. No words could express his disappointment. I felt an urgency to respond to his aching heart.

"Bruno, please be patient. It'll take time for the drugs to work," I said. "I believe tomorrow will be a better day." It was an overly optimistic statement.

"You are right, Dr. Jim. Is too early. I too believe tomorrow is a good day," he said with a smile. Before I had a chance to assess his intentions, he threw his arms around me and hugged me tightly.

"Thank you, Dr. Jim." The giant man released me, then turned and walked away.

I dealt with a tangle of emotions—the uncertainty, the possibility that what we had tried to do for Rani was all for naught and yet, a glimmer of hope that the injections would give this beautiful animal a better quality of life, if only for a while.

I was deep in thought when Marco put a hand on my shoulder. "Don't worry about him. Whatever happens with Rani, Bruno will be okay." He laughed. "Although he is my baby brother, he has always been twice my size. His body is as hard as a rock, but his heart is quite soft. We are so thankful for what you have done for Rani. I have cash in my safe. Please, what do we owe you?"

Rani slowly slipped into her arena, barely touching her left front foot to the ground, and quietly laid down. "Marco, I haven't had this much excitement in a long time," I said. "Please accept what my staff and I have done this morning as our gift to Rani."

He looked at me, then lowered his head to disguise his tears. "I don't know what to say."

I reached out and shook his hand. "If you will be so kind as to let me know how she does, then I'll keep my fingers crossed. To know that she is walking on four feet again will be payment enough."

Suddenly, Marco took a deep breath, as if he had just remembered something important. "Doctor, do you have family?"

"Uh, yes, I do. My wife and I have two young boys."

He held up a finger. "Will you please excuse me for one minute?" He turned and ran toward the line of trailers. In less than a minute, he was back. He held four tickets in his hand.

"It will be an honor for Bruno and me to have you and your family as our guests at tomorrow's show. I will reserve special seats for you," he said proudly.

I took the tickets from his hand and read the bold print: ***Barcini Brothers Circus. Experience the magic of life.***

"Thank you, Marco. My family and I would love to see your show," I said with a broad smile.

Our boys, now five and eight years of age, were ecstatic when I told them of my adventure with the tiger and showed them the tickets.

"Do you think we'll get to pet Rani, Papa?" JT asked.

"No, I don't think so, son. I doubt she'll even be able to perform. Maybe I can talk Bruno into letting us see her after the show."

We woke the next morning to a cold front. The wind blew and the air was chilly—not a favorable day for Rani's foot. Showtime was six o'clock that evening. I wanted to be there early. It was five when we drove into the parking lot. Some of Marco's crew, wearing bright clothes and painted faces, directed traffic. In front of us was an enormous circus tent surrounded by colorful flags that snapped in the breeze.

We followed the signs to the public entrance and the ticket booth. There wasn't a single person waiting in line.

"Do you think we're early enough?" Katy asked in her most facetious voice.

At the entrance to the tent, a man stood behind a podium. He wore a black tuxedo, a starched white shirt, and a black bowtie. It was Bruno, selling tickets. He recognized me, stepped from behind the podium, and threw his arms open.

"Dr. Jim! Is my supreme pleasure to see you. I am such honored that you come to see our show." He threw his arms around me and kissed me on both cheeks, as was the European custom.

It took me a moment to catch my breath. "The honor is entirely ours, Bruno. I'd like you to meet my family," I said. "This is my wife, Katy."

Katy reached out to shake his hand. Bruno bowed, gently cradled Katy's fingers in the tips of his, and kissed the back of her hand. "This is very special, Mrs. Katy, that you come to see our show."

"We wouldn't miss this for the world, Bruno," Katy said. "I'm so pleased to meet you. Jim has told us a lot about you . . . and Rani. My boys have never been to a circus. They are very excited. These are my two sons, JT and Rob."

The boys looked up, in awe of the giant man who stood before them. Bruno gave each of them a firm handshake.

"Hallo, boys," he said. "You look much like," turning first toward me, then toward Katy, "your mother." As well as being courageous, courteous, and compassionate, Bruno was also very diplomatic.

He whistled to someone in the distance. "Dr. Jim, I have reserved special seats for you, Mrs. Katy, and boys."

I was nervous about asking the question, but I just had to know. "How is she doing, Bruno? How is Rani?"

19 – Rani Part II

"She is okay. She is resting well," he said with a smile. A man appeared at Bruno's side. He was muscular, had thick hair, a full beard, and was not quite three feet tall.

"Dr. Jim, this is Venzo. He show your seats," Bruno said. "Perhaps, we talk after show."

We followed Venzo into the tent. It wasn't until we were inside that we realized how spectacular it was. The ground had been carefully raked, not a single visible rock or piece of paper—the result of all the hard work I had witnessed the day before. The outer perimeter was a solid ring of bleachers. A walkway divided the front row from three rows of VIP seats, which in turn, were fronted by wooden blocks that delineated the ring. In the center of the ring was a raised net and high above the net was a high-wire and trapeze swings. The right side of the ring was separated by a giant curtain from what looked like a remaining quarter of the tent.

We followed Venzo past the center of the ring to the far-right side, next to the curtain. Venzo directed us to the front row. "I'll be right back," he said and smiled.

In a matter of minutes, he returned with a tray carrying two bags of popcorn and soft drinks. He handed them to JT and Rob. "Enjoy," he said.

The boys looked at each other with excitement on their faces like two kids on Christmas morning.

"Wow. I've never seen anything like this," Katy said. "Everything is so pristine."

The noise inside the tent became louder as a steady stream of people filed in. As show time approached, I scanned the audience. It was a full house. Excitement and energy filled the air.

Classic circus music blared through huge speakers, strategically mounted on the walls of the tent. The music was suddenly interrupted by a drum roll. The lights dimmed. A man stepped out from behind the curtain and walked to center stage. He wore shiny black pants and boots, a red tuxedo jacket with tails, a white shirt with ruffles complimented by a bowtie that matched his jacket, and a black top-hat. A spotlight shone on him as he picked up a microphone.

"Ladies and gentlemen, welcome to Barcini Brothers Circus!" An enthusiastic round of applause erupted throughout the tent. At first, I wasn't sure about his identity, but the voice was unmistakable. It was Marco. He drew a whistle from his coat pocket and blew it loudly.

Once again, the tent was alive with music. From the far-left side of the tent, the opening procession marched in. JT stepped up onto his seat as I hoisted Rob onto my shoulders.

A group of clowns with painted faces and dressed in loose clothes, raised a cloud of dust with their floppy shoes as they walked between the bleachers and the VIP seats and passed out helium-filled balloons to the kids in the audience. It was an event of grandeur not previously experienced by JT and Rob. Anticipation burned like fire inside of them as one of the clowns approached and handed each of them a balloon. It was then that I noticed the faded, worn material of his costume, the stitching of the tears in his shirt and pants, evidence that this show, however professionally executed, struggled financially.

19 – Rani Part II

The boys saw a completely different picture. Their eyes were fixed, mesmerized by the broad painted smile, the kind eyes with long lashes that reached out and touched their hearts with both sadness and beauty.

A tiny motorized car that looked like a medium-sized cardboard box entered the ring pulling a trailer. A beautiful lady in a sparkly costume followed the car, accompanied by five miniature poodles, all dressed in flashy tutus. Four little people stepped out of the car. One retrieved bowling pins from the trailer while another, neon rings. They performed an amazing juggling act. The other two took baskets full of little bags of peanuts and tossed them into the crowd. Simultaneously, the lady wearing the sparkles directed the poodles through a series of acrobatic stunts. The crowd cheered.

The first act ended and the ring was cleared of dogs and debris. Two of the clowns began a brilliant comedy act. The first clown dropped a lit firecracker into the second clown's pants. After the firecracker exploded, the second clown took his revenge. He picked up a bucket full of water, chased the first clown into the audience, and heaved the contents into the middle of the crowd. The people screamed and covered their faces only to be surprised—the bucket was full of confetti. JT and Rob laughed so loud, I felt certain that their bellies must hurt.

Marco was the perfect ringmaster. He entertained the crowd as each act finished and cleaned up in preparation for the next.

The boys stared, clapped, and gasped. The high-wire and trapeze artists performed their shows with the most exciting and nerve-racking stunts I had ever seen. It was a fantastic show, full of color, excitement, suspense, drama, and laughter.

Once again, the spotlight shined on Marco as he walked to center ring. With his chin held high, he surveyed the crowd.

"Ladies and gentlemen. On behalf of everyone at Barcini Brothers Circus, I wish to thank you for spending this evening with us. We hope that you have enjoyed our show." The crowd cried out for more. "Before you leave us tonight, I am thrilled to present to you, one more member of our family." He extended his hand toward the curtain at the right side of the ring.

"Ladies and gentlemen, meet Rani!"

The curtain was drawn revealing Rani's arena. I was stunned. The last thing I had expected was for Rani to make an appearance.

"Look, Papa!" JT yelled, as he pulled on my shirt sleeve. "It's Rani!"

Rob jumped up and down. "Rani, Papa, Rani!"

The steel bars were no more than ten feet from our "special seats." A jig-saw puzzle of thick red, white, and blue colored rubber mats covered the ground inside the circle. In the center of the steel ring, arms crossed, feet apart, chin high, Bruno stood tall and took a formal bow. He wore a tight leotard that covered his entire body from his ankles and wrists up to his neck. It was rippled with orange stripes interrupted by thin black lines and patches of white. He was barefoot. He could easily have passed for Rani's twin brother. Next to him, her head held high, Rani let out a roar that was both exciting and spine tingling. The crowd responded with a roar of our own.

19 – Rani Part II

Bruno slowly walked to the edge of the arena. He carried nothing, not a chair nor a whip, nor even a cane. He whispered something to Rani and gestured toward a group of wooden obstacles that had been placed in the center of the ring. Without hesitation, Rani stood and walked to the first obstacle. She didn't limp. I couldn't believe it. I concentrated on her left front leg as she trotted up the first obstacle, a series of steps, and down the other side. She jumped onto a giant cylinder, balanced on it as it rolled ten feet, then jumped off and landed gracefully on all four feet.

I suddenly realized I was holding my breath. I was overwhelmed with emotion. Rani jumped through several steel hoops, returned to the center of the ring, and sat down, to the deafening cheers of the crowd. Bruno knelt next to her, draped his arms around her neck and laid his cheek against hers. The crowd went wild. They clapped, they yelled, and they whistled. JT and Rob stood motionless, eyes and mouths wide open. The wide smile on Katy's face confirmed both the depth and the warmth of the experience.

Bruno slowly rose to his feet, pointed to the edge of the arena, and whispered something to Rani, who trotted toward the steel bars and then began to circle as she hugged the inner perimeter of the arena. The brilliant colors of her coat shimmered like glass under the bright lights. The muscles of her shoulders, back and hips moved in synchrony with the ease and power of a well-oiled machine. Each time she approached the center ring, she raised her head high and looked into the crowd, no tricks necessary to show off her beauty.

Bruno kept his eyes on her as she went around, again and again. Slowly, she increased her pace. Each time she circled to our side of the arena, Bruno looked in our direction and smiled. He clapped once, then twice. Rani began to prance. The rhythm of her step was slow at first, one, two, one, two. The rhythm picked up, one, two, one, two. The crowd quickly found the rhythm and joined in as they clapped, one, two, one, two. Rani threw her chin up and roared. She held her head and chest high. With every step, each foot was raised into the air, projected forward horizontally, and stamped to the ground in perfect time to the clapping of hundreds of pairs of hands. From the last row of bleachers forward, every person in the tent rose from his or her seat. They clapped, stomped their feet, and chanted, "RA-NI, RA-NI, RA-NI."

Rani looked deep into the audience and pranced, and pranced, as if to assure us, one and all, that life . . . is magical.

Chapter 20
TIME TO SAY GOODBYE

It was perhaps the greatest journey of my life, often challenging and exhausting, but always rewarding. It started in 1978 when I was accepted to the veterinary school at Texas A&M University, and it spanned more than three decades. With the never-ending love and support of my wife, Katy, I managed the difficult times, like fourteen years of working Sundays at the sale barn, and I relished the best of times, like watching our boys, JT and Rob, grow into young men. I had the good fortune of having the greatest partner anyone could have asked for in Mike and exceptional staff members like Santiago, Roseann, and Christine. Along my journey, I made great friends and had wonderful clients like Ruth Simpson and Ben Garner. I experienced memorable occasions like the night that Jay and I lit up the skies of southeastern New Mexico with a fireworks display that went awry. Not all my friends were human. Some were furry, others feathered, and they walked barefoot. They were the reason I got up every morning. Some were loving, like Hershey and Placido, others were stubborn, like Flossy and Banjo, and still others were dangerous, like Big Bird and Rani. They were all special to their owners and they became special to me. Like everything in life, the time comes when one reaches the end of the journey and I had arrived at mine.

It was the end of another long day. Mike and I sat at our desks and enjoyed the peace and quiet. Then he cleared his throat and sighed.

"I think it's time for me to cash out, Jim," he said.

"What are you talking about?" I wasn't completely surprised by his remark. Mike had just celebrated his 67th birthday and I was a month away from my 58th. Many times, we had talked about calling it quits. I had made it clear to Mike that I wasn't interested in buying his share of the practice. What we had started together, poured our hearts and souls into building together, we decided to give up together.

"I'm tired," Mike said. "It's been a long, hard road. Sure would like to finish on top."

For thirty years, Mike had been my brother. Our partnership worked for the same reason our marriages did—compromise, patience, respect, and love. It hadn't been without sacrifice. In the early years, we had occasionally not written ourselves a paycheck in order to pay the bills. For fourteen years, we gave up our Sundays with our families to work at the sale barn just to make ends meet. In the years that followed, we turned our two-doctor practice into a hospital with a staff of twenty employees and five doctors.

We developed and held steadfast to a strict policy—If somebody called us with an emergency, no matter who or what time of day or night, we responded. Mike had a favorite saying, "If we had wanted to be millionaires and get a good night's sleep, we'd have gone to law school."

20 – *Time to Say Goodbye*

"I'm ready if you are. Where do we start?" I asked.

"Well, that corporate bunch is still biting at the bit to buy us out. They're not my first choice, but I'm not sure we have another option," he replied.

Sadly, Mike was right. All our associates were young, recent graduates with huge student debts. One of them made a bold attempt to buy the practice, but our client base had grown to the point that banks were not willing to make a loan of that magnitude to an individual with existing debt.

Six months later, in February of 2012, we sold our practice to a corporation. The agreement was for Mike and me to continue to work for them for the following two years. In return, they agreed to let us continue to practice just like we always had. The truth was, we knew better.

Two weeks into my new life as an employee of the corporation, I walked in the front door of our house, through the hallway to the kitchen, and slammed my car keys on the counter.

"Whoa! This doesn't sound very good," Katy said.

I drew a deep breath and expelled it without any attempt to hide my exasperation. "You know what they want me to do now?"

"I assume 'they' are your new employers? No. Tell me. What do they want you to do now?" She was unsure whether to frown or smile.

"They want me to check my e-mails twice a day. Can you believe that? Who the hell has time to be checking their e-mails twice a day?"

"Time is the least of your problems, sweetie," she said with a smile. "You don't know what e-mail is, much less how to get online and check it."

"Well, yeah, but they don't know that."

She cleared her throat. "What are you going to do?"

"Haven't got a clue. Ignore them, I guess."

"Let me talk to Roseann," she said. "I bet she'll be willing to screen them for you. If she finds anything important enough to warrant your attention, she can fill you in. What do you think?"

Mike and I had insisted that Roseann be promoted from receptionist to hospital manager. Her new position meant a significant increase in salary and she earned it with extensive training, daily calls to the corporate office, weekly conference calls, and a ton of red tape that kept us in compliance with the corporation's wishes.

I pretended to give Katy's idea careful thought. "Yeah. Good idea." I sighed. "There's more."

"Oh, yeah," she said casually with a subtle grin.

"They're giving me six weeks' vacation a year."

"What? Six weeks of vacation? You've never taken six weeks off in the same year since the day we moved here," she said. She gave me a broad smile.

"Yeah, but they want me to request all vacation in writing, a minimum of six weeks in advance. Is that crazy or what?"

"Have you forgotten who you're talking to? I worked for the U.S. government for thirteen years. Welcome to the real world, pal." She

20 – Time to Say Goodbye

laughed, then she put her arm around my neck and pulled my head next to hers. "What's really wrong?" she whispered.

I shook my head and fought back tears. "I don't know. I feel like a traitor, like I've sold out my staff and clients. A lot of people have depended on me for lots of years, sweetie. How do I say to them, *'Sorry, but I'm gone?'*" She ran her fingers through my hair and gently kissed me on the forehead.

"You've paid your dues, over and over again. You're tired—really tired. I can see it," she said as she stared into my eyes. "They'll understand and they'll be okay . . . and so will you."

She was right. It was time for me to call it quits, but it took some time before I was able to accept the fact. It was a steep cliff from where I had fallen—half owner of a successful veterinary practice to a mere corporate employee. It was by choice, but it was still a difficult pill to swallow.

There was an indisputable rule in corporate medicine, *charge for everything you do.* That meant *everything* to them. It was a rule that, at times, I found difficult to comply with.

For years, part of my treatment protocol for a dog with a bad ear infection included weekly follow-up exams until I was satisfied that the ear was completely free of infection. Some cases required five or six quick visits to make sure my client was complying with my instructions and the ear was improving. As incentive to make sure I got those follow-ups, I only charged for the initial exam. Subsequent visits were free except for the cost of any medication. It was perhaps not the best business practice in the short term, but satisfied clients make loyal clients.

Now I was told I couldn't operate in that manner, but then, I didn't always do what I was told. Unfortunately, my stubbornness put our receptionists and Roseann in a difficult position. They had to explain the "no charge" exams in the accounting records. Although I never knew for sure, I suspected some of my recheck exams never got entered into the computer records. As long as we kept revenues up, which we did, the corporation was satisfied with our performance.

That first year passed in the blink of an eye. Then, Pop, Katy's dad, passed away. Katy's mom lived in Las Cruces, 180 miles away, was in good health, and sharp as a tack, but Katy felt an urgency to be closer to her. We decided the time had come to plan our move across the mountains to Las Cruces.

I was six months from my final day in Roswell when I began hearing the same question almost daily.

"Dr. Humphreys, I heard a rumor yesterday," Mrs. Romero said.

"What are you talking about, Leigh Ann?" I asked as if I didn't know.

"Are you really leaving?" she asked.

I closed my eyes and sighed. "Yeah. The end of June."

"What am I supposed to do? Who's going to take care of Jack?"

The knot in my throat tightened. A forced smile seemed so artificial, and yet, so necessary. "Jack is gonna be just fine, Leigh Ann. We're interviewing candidates to replace me right now. It'll be okay. I promise."

20 – Time to Say Goodbye

"Maybe I could come see you at your new hospital," she said.

"I'm not going to have a new hospital, Leigh Ann. I'm sorta retiring. I'm thinking of working part-time for an old friend of mine. His clinic is four hours from here."

I felt horrible. She smiled, but I could tell she was upset. I had taken care of Jack, a vivacious Miniature Schnauzer, from the time he was a pup. Leigh Ann and I had been through several dog crises together throughout the years. I knew how she felt. I had also placed my trust in the hands of several family physicians over the years only to see them retire. My son, Rob, said it best when he became aware that, after our move, he would no longer return to what had always been his home—"Change is the pits."

The closer I got to my departure date, the more loose ends I realized I still had to tie up. Above my desk was a bookshelf with several rows of big, thick, heavy textbooks. "You're welcome to any or all of these books," I told the youngest of my associates one morning.

She looked at me with a strange sneer. "You're kidding me, right?"

"No, I'm serious. I don't think I'll be needing them anymore." I pulled one off the shelf and opened it. "There's some great stuff in this one," I said.

She shook her head and laughed. "Jim, you're such a dinosaur. I have the updated version of that book right here in my phone."

"Really? Well, my phone isn't as smart as yours. I wonder if the library might want them."

As it turned out, the library didn't want any of them either—they went into the dumpster. Time caught up with me quickly. Before I knew it, June had arrived, and my last day was a month away.

It was a busy Tuesday morning. After a short break for lunch, I walked past our three primary exam rooms. Each door had a patient record attached and the name of the doctor each client had requested. All three doors had my name on them. I rushed down the hallway to Roseann's office. "What the heck is going on, Roseann?" I asked.

"What do you mean, sir?" she asked with a puzzled look.

"They scheduled three appointments for me all at the same time. They know better than that," I said with impatience.

"Dr. Humphreys, with one exception, everybody who's coming in this afternoon has an appointment to see you. It was the only way to accommodate everybody," Roseann said calmly. "We did the same thing for Dr. Mike's favorite clients yesterday afternoon. Today is your day."

I was dumbfounded for a moment. "You know how I hate to keep people waiting, Roseann," I said, somewhat irritated. "I'll do what I can, but that third client may be sitting there for a while."

"We explained that to them, Dr. Humphreys. They're all okay with it," she said with a compassionate voice. "Ruth Simpson got here just after you left for lunch. You may want to see her first."

"What's the matter with Bingo?" I asked.

"I'm not sure, sir."

Bingo was Ruth Simpson's Blue Heeler. Even though he guarded Ruth's pig farm with tenacity, Bingo was an incredibly sweet dog. "Hi,

20 – Time to Say Goodbye

Ruth," I said as I walked into the exam room and gave her a big hug. Then I looked around the room. "Where's Bingo?"

"Bingo's fine, Jim. I didn't bring him." I was confused. Then I saw a tear slowly slide down her cheek. "I just needed to say goodbye one last time," Ruth said. "Gonna miss you something awful."

I felt a tightening in my chest. "I'm going to miss you too, Ruth. Wish I could take you, Bingo, and Rosebud with me." I struggled with my words. "Mike and I have interviewed some sharp young doctors. They'll take good care of you. I promise." I wiped the tears from my face and chuckled. "If they don't, you call me and I'll come back here and beat them with a stick."

We reminisced for some time. Ruth reminded me of the night I showed up at her barn to deliver Rosebud's babies with Rob, still in a diaper. "You broke that baby boy in the hard way that night, Jim." We both laughed, then we cried, hugged, and she left. Each successive exam room held the same story—my client without their dog or cat, a period of reminiscence, hugs, and a final farewell.

By late afternoon, I was spent. My heart ached and my eyes had cried enough tears to fill a lake. "How am I gonna get away with this, Roseann? I can't charge these people for coming to say goodbye. I know every one of them will gladly pay for an office visit, but I just can't do it."

"Don't worry about it, Dr. Humphreys. It's been taken care of," she said and winked.

On the 30th of June, I took a cardboard box to work. I emptied the drawers of my desk, took down my collection of pictures of my boys, staff, clients, and patients, and gathered the last of my junk. I had already decided that staying the entire day was more than I could handle and so, one by one, I hugged each of my staff, wished them well, and gave my eternal thanks for all they had done to make our hospital the finest in New Mexico.

"You're the best, Dr. Humphreys," Roseann said.

I was emotionally drained, but my last words were important to me. "Don't know about that. What I do know is, you're the one who brings out the best in all of us, Roseann. You're the heart of this hospital . . . don't ever forget that."

That evening, Katy and I dined with Mike and Dianne at their home. "We had a pretty good run, Jim," Mike said. "Have any regrets?"

"Sure I do, but not enough to change my mind. It was time. How about you?" I asked. "Was our timing right?"

"Yeah, it was, but I'm sure going to miss my partner. When are you guys leaving?" he asked.

"We'll take the first load next week. I left a few things at Jay's. We'll be back for them later," I replied.

It was a perfect evening. We reminisced about our thirty-three years together. Mike talked solemnly about the abuse we had both endured at the hands of Dr. T and how fortunate we were to have stuck it out together. I reminded him of the rabies suspect and the horse's head that we lost. He reflected on fourteen long years of Sundays at the sale barn listening to Stan. We talked about our great employees—Brenda, Jon Boy, Santiago, Christine, Roseann, and all the rest. We

20 – Time to Say Goodbye

recalled the annual Christmas gift exchanges in front of a roaring fire and gave thanks for the enduring friendship among our kids. We laughed and we cried. As we faced the end, we hugged each other tightly and said goodbye.

****

Two weeks later, Katy and I stood under the cover of Jay's new workshop and watched the rain come down. Jay had built a shop to keep all his tractors and farm equipment out of the weather. The building looked like a hanger, large enough to house a 747 jetliner. The last of our possessions were neatly packed in a U-Haul trailer. Katy and Carrie hugged and bid their farewells.

"Can't believe you're actually doing this, Jim. Just doesn't seem right," Jay said.

"Oh, I guess we all have our own stories to play out, Jay. Look at you. A California hippie turned New Mexico farmer-rancher? Pretty crazy."

"I remember that first day we met," Jay said. "I sold you a really ugly piece of carpet, wound up taking it home for you, and got a plate of nachos and a beer for my trouble."

I laughed. "Yeah. It's kind of ironic, isn't it?"

"How's that?" he asked.

"You were the first person I said *hi* to when I rolled into this town. The first guy I shook hands with. Thirty-three years later, I'm about to roll out of this town and you're the last person I'll say *goodbye* to and the last hand I'll shake." I sighed sadly.

"Handshake, my ass. Give me a hug," he said with open arms. "Then get the hell out of here before I start to cry."

It was a long, tight, meaningful embrace. He was tougher than I was. I just couldn't hold back the tears.

"You know what, Jay? I think instead of saying goodbye, I'm gonna leave it at, see ya."

"Yeah. I like that, Jim . . . see ya."

EPILOGUE

MY FRIENDS WALK BAREFOOT

Epilogue

Ysleta Independent School District
Central Office
El Paso, Texas
March 19, 2022

The boys and girls of the Eastwood Knolls Middle School Band marched off the stage in a well-disciplined and quiet manner that would make any military commander proud. They wore their sharp uniform of black pants, white shirts, blue vests, and matching blue bowties. The combination of seventh and eighth graders had just performed three musical pieces before a panel of judges. They were tough judges—with acute ears for musical notes and errors that only true professional musicians could hear. This was the yearly evaluation of the school bands in the Ysleta School District.

The band marched to the Sight Reading Room where three more judges waited for them. Each band member was handed new music sheets, which they had never seen or practiced. The Eastwood Knolls Band had just performed and they were about to do it again, only this time, they had seven minutes to study the new sheets and together, transform those notes into a melodic sound called music.

Each judge evaluated the band's performance with a score of five to one—*five* was the lowest score and *one* meant a superior performance. To achieve a unanimous score of *ones* from all judges required true excellence. It was called "Sweepstakes."

Katy and I stood outside the Sight Reading Room and listened. Marty Olivas, a professional musician and the Director of Fine Arts for the district, also waited outside the room in anticipation of the band's performance and scores. He asked if we wanted to sneak in, but the room was much smaller than the auditorium in which they had just played and we dared not make the band any more nervous.

"That was big boy music they just played," Marty said. "That's music even some high school band directors won't touch."

Suddenly, the first notes penetrated through the door and walls as the band began to play the piece they had just received. The hallway was soon filled with a beautiful melody. It was perfect, I thought.

A young lady who sat behind the information desk in the hallway said, "Wow! They sound awesome. Who's their band director?"

"His name is JT . . . He's my son," I said proudly as I struggled to hold back the tears.

Marty Olivas had hired JT seven years earlier. "Hiring JT was one of the best decisions I ever made," he said.

Later that evening, we received a phone call. It was that boy who was once my loyal assistant and braved the bloody laceration on Daisy's back.

"We got Sweepstakes," he said proudly. "All *ones*!"

Epilogue

Ball Arena
Denver, Colorado
February 16, 2022

The evening was energized with excitement and the venue filled with the clamor of anxious fans. Katy and I sat close to the stage. The lights dimmed, and then, the concert hall went completely dark. A sudden surge of applause and loud cheering from the crowd filled the arena. The first chords of instrumental music began and resonated in a soft melody. My throat tightened and my eyes welled. I was overcome with emotion. In the beam of a single spotlight, the six-time Grammy award winner appeared. Kacey Musgraves stood against the backdrop of blues and purples and began to sing "Star Crossed" in her soft and unique voice.

The multi-color lights slowly lit the stage and revealed her band, the lead guitar player on the right side, the bass player in the middle, and in the forefront, on the left side of the stage was the drummer—our son, Rob, the little boy who once sat in a barn, his back against a hay bale, surrounded by baby pigs trying to nurse from his toes, and wearing nothing more than a diaper.

Funny how things turn out.